Sobriety

by Lane Kennedy and Tamar Medford

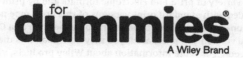

for **dummies®**

A Wiley Brand

Sobriety For Dummies®

Published by: **John Wiley & Sons, Inc.,** 111 River Street, Hoboken, NJ 07030-5774, www.wiley.com

Copyright © 2025 by John Wiley & Sons, Inc., Hoboken, New Jersey

Media and software compilation copyright © 2025 by John Wiley & Sons, Inc. All rights reserved.

Published simultaneously in Canada

For general information on our other products and services, please contact our Customer Care Department within the U.S. at 877-762-2974, outside the U.S. at 317-572-3993, or fax 317-572-4002. For technical support, please visit www.wiley.com/techsupport.

Wiley publishes in a variety of print and electronic formats and by print-on-demand. Some material included with standard print versions of this book may not be included in e-books or in print-on-demand. If this book refers to media such as a CD or DVD that is not included in the version you purchased, you may download this material at http://booksupport.wiley.com. For more information about Wiley products, visit www.wiley.com.

Library of Congress Control Number: 2024943444

ISBN 978-1-394-25416-3 (pbk); ISBN 978-1-394-25417-0 (ebk); ISBN 978-1-394-25418-7 (ebk)

SKY10081751_081024

Table of Contents

CHAPTER 8: **Embracing Mental, Physical, and Emotional Well-Being** 157

CHAPTER 9: **Finding Your Purpose and Joy** 195

Introduction

L iving a sober life is more than just a cessation of alcohol; it's a profound and transformative experience. Whether you've grappled with alcoholism yourself or supported a loved one through their recovery, understanding the nuances of addiction and the journey to a life of recovery is essential. This book aims to guide you through the many layers of sobriety, offering practical advice, emotional support, and abundant knowledge to help you flourish in your journey to long-term recovery.

Sobriety transcends mere abstinence. It's about embracing an entirely new way of living. It's about finding clarity amid the chaos, healing old wounds, and envisioning a future filled with purpose and joy. The road to long-term sobriety is undeniably challenging and fraught with emotional, physical, and psychological obstacles. It's called living life. Yet, this journey can be incredibly rewarding with the right tools and support. This book is designed to be your steadfast companion, providing the insights and guidance you need to confidently navigate each step.

The journey of long-term recovery is one of self-discovery and transformation. It asks you to uncover the underlying causes of your addiction and recognize the sparks (in the context of this book, a "spark" refers to a moment or situation that ignites a response challenging your commitment to sobriety) that leads to substance use, and developing strategies to overcome these challenges. In this book, we will explore the complex interplay of genetics, your brain, environment, and spirituality in addiction, offering a comprehensive approach to recovery. Understanding these dimensions will give you a deeper insight into yourself and what influences your sober life.

A crucial aspect of recovery is building a supportive network. Sobriety is not an endeavor to be undertaken alone or to live in a vacuum. Recovery thrives on the collective efforts of friends, family, and support groups. This book provides practical advice on cultivating a strong support system, navigating social settings, and building meaningful connections that foster long-term sobriety. By the end of this book, you will have the knowledge and tools you need to succeed and thrive in your sober lifestyle, overcoming obstacles and celebrating the joy of a life free from addiction.

Each chapter of this book explores a specific aspect of sobriety. From understanding the nature of alcoholism to developing life-long recovery strategies, you will find valuable information designed to support you at every stage of your journey. Approach this material with an open mind and a willingness to reflect on your experiences. As you align your actions with your sobriety goals, you will witness the powerful impact of this journey and discover the clear, fulfilling life that awaits you.

About This Book

This book serves as a comprehensive guide to sobriety, from understanding the mental illness named *alcoholism* to cultivating long-term recovery strategies for life. It covers genetic, environmental, and spiritual influences while also offering practical advice for creating a genuine and fulfilling sober lifestyle.

You'll discover the emotional challenges of recovery, learn how to navigate social situations and maintain your overall well-being. The book also addresses overcoming obstacles, managing relapse, and creating a long-term foundation platform for sustained sobriety. The goal is to help you recognize the power of sobriety, understand the various facets of recovery, and maintain a fulfilling, sober life.

The point of this book is to help you become conscious of the power of sobriety. To this end, we will provide you with the means of identifying and understanding the various aspects of recovery and offer tips for maintaining a long-term recovery.

Conventions Used in This Book

To help you navigate through this book, I use the following conventions:

>> *Italic* is used to emphasize and highlight new words or defined terms.

>> **Boldfaced** text indicates keywords in bulleted lists or the action part of numbered steps.

>> Monofont is used for web addresses.

>> Sidebars, which look like text enclosed in a shaded gray box, consist of information that's interesting to know but not necessarily critical to your understanding of the chapter or section topic. We also included real stories from people who have made the sobriety journey.

Foolish Assumptions

We assume that you

>> Are interested in sobriety and know a little bit about the subject

>> Want to improve your understanding of addiction and recovery

>> Are willing to reflect and respond as you read each chapter

>> Have a desire to live in or support someone in long-term recovery from alcoholism

How This Book Is Organized

Throughout this book, you'll have the opportunity to learn about the intricate aspects of sobriety. You'll start by understanding the nuances of alcoholism and addiction, then move on to uncover effective strategies for long-term recovery. In each section, you'll find practical advice on navigating social situations, building emotional resilience, and creating a personalized recovery plan.

Each section is designed to meet you where you are in your recovery journey, providing you with the tools and knowledge you need to thrive in sobriety.

Part I: From Chaos to Clarity: Stepping Into Sobriety

This part introduces the concepts of alcoholism and sobriety, helping you understand the growth of addiction, the differences between heavy drinking and alcoholism, and the importance of embracing sobriety.

Part II: Decoding the Elements of Addiction: Genetics, Environment, and Spiritual Dynamics

In this part, you explore the genetic and environmental factors that contribute to addiction. You will also learn about the impact of family dynamics, the spiritual dimension of recovery, and how to navigate these elements on your path to long-term recovery.

Part III: Living (and Loving) a Sober Lifestyle

This part provides practical advice on building a solid foundation for a sober lifestyle, from establishing a strong support system to nurturing mental, physical, and emotional well-being. You will find tools that will support your sober lifestyle.

Part IV: Overcoming Challenges and Thriving in Sobriety

Here, you'll learn how to handle challenges and potential relapses. The chapters in this part offer strategies for coping with triggers, rebuilding trust within the family and developing a career in sobriety.

Part V: The Road to Long-Term Sobriety

Part five focuses on sustaining long-term sobriety. You'll discover how to create a sustainable, sober-friendly routine, develop coping mechanisms, and build resilience for lasting recovery.

Part VI: The Part of Tens

If you prefer easily accessible information, this part is for you. In Parts of Ten, you will practical tips and strategies, such as ten ways to discover your purpose in sobriety and ten ways to achieve long-term recovery.

Icons Used in This Book

For sharpening your thinking and focusing your attention, let these icons be your guide:

REMEMBER

This icon underscores a valuable point to keep in mind.

TIP

These are practical and immediate remedies for becoming a skilled and confident body language practitioner.

WARNING

This icon highlights potentially awkward situations to avoid.

Beyond the Book

Find out more about Sobriety for Dummies by checking out the bonus content at www.dummies.com.

You can locate the book's Cheat Sheet at, www.dummies.com. Type "Sobriety For Dummies Cheat Sheet" in the search box. There you'll find handy hints and tips.

We've also included three full chapters that you can find on the Dummies website:

>> Unraveling the Myths: Dispelling Common Misconceptions about Sobriety

>> Nature Versus Nurture in Family Relations

>> Building a Solid Foundation

Where to Go from Here

Although all the material in this book is designed to support you in your journey to sobriety, not all the information may be pertinent to your specific needs or interests. Read what you want, when you want. You don't have to read the book in any specific order, nor is there a sell-by date for covering the material.

If you're interested in understanding alcoholism, begin with Part I. If you're seeking strategies for overcoming challenges in sobriety, have a look at Part IV. If you're curious about building a solid foundation for a sober lifestyle, turn to Part III. And if you want to develop long-term recovery strategies, go to Part V.

Now, turn to a page, chapter, or section that interests you and begin reading. We hope you take away something useful and have fun in the process.

1

From Chaos to Clarity: Stepping Into Sobriety

Chapter **1**

The Basics of Sobriety

Welcome to a journey of sustained recovery and personal growth. This book is dedicated to achieving sobriety, maintaining it for the long haul, and doing so with joy! While many people manage to stop drinking, the challenge of staying sober is an enduring one. It *requires* ongoing effort, resilience, and a deep understanding of the complexities of your addiction. Our goal is to provide you with the knowledge and tools necessary to support an evolving, sober life, fully embracing the continuous recovery process; it doesn't end.

In this chapter, we will uncover the intricacies of alcoholism, sobriety, and recovery. You will gain insights into the nature of alcoholism, its far-reaching impacts, and the critical steps needed to build and sustain a happy, sober lifestyle. We will explore the differences between heavy drinking and alcoholism, examine the rising tide of alcohol addiction, and understand the phenomenon of cross-addiction. By understanding these concepts, you can navigate your recovery journey more effectively, develop robust coping strategies, and cultivate a fulfilling, alcohol-free life. Welcome to your journey of lifelong recovery.

Understanding Sobriety and Alcoholism

Alcoholism is a complex condition that goes beyond mere over-indulgence in alcohol; it's a serious disorder, a mental illness that affects both the mind and body. Individuals struggling with alcoholism often face an intense compulsion to drink, losing the ability to regulate their consumption despite knowing the harmful consequences. This disorder impacts not only the physical health of the individual but also their mental well-being and social relationships.

Sobriety, on the other hand, is not just about abstaining from alcohol but involves a transformative journey toward reclaiming one's life and health. It can be beneficial to understand the understanding the root causes of your addiction while developing coping mechanisms and building a support network to maintain a fulfilling, alcohol-free life. Recognizing these elements is crucial in addressing alcoholism effectively and compassionately, paving the way for more effective interventions and lasting recovery.

What is alcoholism?

Alcoholism, also known as alcohol use disorder, is a chronic disease characterized by an inability to control your drinking despite negative consequences. It is recognized by the *Diagnostic and Statistical Manual of Mental Disorders* (DSM) as a mental disorder, and it encompasses a range of physical, mental, and social symptoms. According to physician and addiction expert Gabor Maté, addiction is often rooted in trauma and a lack of emotional connection, making it a multifaceted issue that requires a comprehensive approach to treatment and recovery.

Understanding the complexity of alcoholism involves recognizing its diverse manifestations, which can vary significantly from person to person. Physically, you may experience intense cravings for alcohol, increased tolerance resulting in the need for more alcohol to achieve the same effects, and withdrawal symptoms when you try to reduce or stop drinking. Mentally, alcoholism can lead to distorted thinking patterns, reduced cognitive functions, and emotional instability. Socially, the disorder can cause alienation from family and friends, job loss, and legal issues, among other adverse outcomes.

Importantly, the roots of alcoholism often lie in deeper psychological factors. As noted by Gabor Maté, many individuals struggling with addiction have histories of trauma, adverse childhood experiences, or unresolved emotional pain. The drinking becomes a misguided attempt to self-medicate or cope with these underlying issues. Consequently, for a successful recovery, it is essential to address not only the physical dependence on alcohol but also the emotional and psychological wounds that fuel the addiction.

REMEMBER

Alcoholism, or alcohol use disorder, is a chronic disease characterized by an inability to control drinking despite negative consequences. Recognized as a mental disorder by the DSM, it affects you physically, mentally, and socially. Effective recovery requires a comprehensive approach that addresses both physical dependence and underlying psychological issues, using resources like rehab centers, support groups, counseling, and hotlines.

This comprehensive approach to treatment must include various resources and support systems. Rehabilitation centers can offer structured environments to detoxify and begin healing, while support groups like Alcoholics Anonymous provide communal support and accountability. Counseling is crucial for delving into the psychological aspects of addiction, allowing you to work through trauma and build healthier coping mechanisms. Additionally, hotlines and other immediate support resources can offer critical assistance during moments of crisis. By recognizing alcoholism as a multifaceted disorder, you can seek a more holistic recovery, focusing on physical sobriety and emotional and psychological well-being.

Growth of alcoholism and addiction

Alcoholism and addiction are increasingly common issues worldwide, driven by factors like social normalization, isolation, glorification of alcohol use, and underlying mental health challenges. This growing trend highlights the need to address addiction not just as a personal struggle but as a significant public health issue.

Cultural attitudes play a significant role in the normalization of drinking and drug use. Society often portrays these behaviors as acceptable or even desirable. Media and advertising further glamorize alcohol consumption, making it seem like an essential part of socializing, celebrating, or coping with life's challenges. This widespread acceptance can obscure the dangers of substance use, making it harder for individuals to see when they are developing a problem. By understanding these influences, we can better address the complexities of addiction and work toward effective solutions.

TIP

Recognize that social normalization, media glamorization, and underlying mental health issues contribute significantly to the rise in alcoholism and addiction. Addressing these influences is crucial for effective prevention and recovery. Comprehensive treatment plans should integrate both mental health and addiction services to provide holistic support.

The glorification of alcohol use, in particular, creates a slippery slope where occasional indulgence can seamlessly transition into habitual consumption. High-profile personalities and influencers frequently share posts and stories featuring alcohol, often without showcasing the potential negative consequences. This selective visibility can foster an environment where heavy drinking is seen as stylish or sophisticated rather than a potential pathway to addiction. Moreover, societies where binge drinking is a common pastime may inadvertently encourage individuals to consume larger quantities of alcohol more frequently, increasing the risk of developing addiction.

Underlying mental health issues are another significant factor in the rising rates of alcoholism and addiction. Mental health disorders such as depression, anxiety, and trauma often co-occur with substance use disorders, as individuals may turn to alcohol or drugs as a form of self-medication. This co-occurrence complicates the recovery process, as addressing one issue without considering the other can lead to incomplete treatment and eventual relapse. Thus, comprehensive treatment plans that integrate mental health and addiction services are essential. The increasing incidence of co-occurring disorders highlights the necessity for interventions that address the root causes of addiction, promote mental well-being, and provide long-term support.

Heavy drinker versus alcoholic

Understanding the difference between a heavy drinker and an alcoholic is essential for identifying the severity of an alcohol use issue. A heavy drinker consumes large amounts of alcohol in a short period or regularly but may not be dependent on it. In contrast, an alcoholic shows compulsive behavior and dependence, continuing to consume alcohol despite adverse consequences. Recognizing these distinctions helps in tailoring the appropriate treatment and support for each individual, acknowledging the complex nature of alcohol use disorders.

When distinguishing between a heavy drinker and an alcoholic, it is crucial to look beyond the quantity of alcohol consumed and focus on the underlying patterns and motivations. A heavy drinker may participate in binge drinking or frequent drinking sessions but can retain control over their consumption. They may even be capable of setting limits, refraining from drinking when needed, and not experiencing severe withdrawal symptoms. However, this pattern of behavior can still lead to significant health risks, both physically and socially, and may serve as a precursor to more severe alcohol-related issues.

An alcoholic, on the other hand, exhibits a chronic inability to control their drinking despite negative impacts on their life. This dependency is marked by a compulsive urge to consume alcohol, leading to repeated and often unsuccessful attempts to cut down or quit. Alcoholism is recognized as a mental disorder by the DSM, highlighting the intricate interplay between genetics, trauma, mental health, and behavioral factors. Symptoms of alcoholism can include cravings, loss of control, physical dependence, and an increased tolerance, where more alcohol is needed to achieve the same effects. These symptoms often result in a decline in physical well-being and disrupt personal and professional relationships.

Understanding the distinction between a heavy drinker and an alcoholic is key to identifying the severity of an alcohol use issue. A heavy drinker consumes large amounts of alcohol regularly but may not be dependent, while an alcoholic exhibits compulsive behavior and dependence despite adverse consequences. Recognizing these differences helps tailor appropriate treatments — educational programs and lifestyle changes for heavy drinkers, and comprehensive interventions like rehab and counseling for alcoholics. This nuanced approach ensures each individual receives the specific support they need.

Cross-addictions

Cross-addiction occurs when individuals develop a new addiction to another substance or behavior after recovering from a previous one. This phenomenon highlights the importance of a holistic approach to recovery, addressing the root causes of addiction and promoting whole-body wellness. By understanding cross-addictions, you can better navigate your recovery journey, implement effective coping strategies, and cultivate a lifestyle that supports long-term sobriety and personal growth.

Identifying potential cross-addictions

Understanding and identifying cross-addictions is an essential part of your recovery journey. This exercise is designed to help you recognize whether you may be experiencing or at risk for cross-addiction. Set aside some quiet time to reflect on the questions below and answer them as honestly as possible while following these steps.

1. **Self-assessment questions.**

   - **Patterns and behaviors:** Have you noticed yourself engaging in any new compulsive behaviors since beginning your recovery? (These might include excessive shopping, gambling, eating, and so on.) Do you find yourself relying on any new substances to cope with stress or emotions (such as caffeine, nicotine, prescription drugs, and the like)?

- **Emotional response:** Do you experience similar emotional highs or lows with your new behavior or substance as you did with your previous addiction? Are you using this new behavior or substance to escape reality, numb emotions, or cope with underlying issues?

- **Impact on life:** Is this new behavior or substance affecting your daily life, relationships, work, or overall well-being? Do you feel a loss of control over this new behavior or substance, similar to your previous addiction?

- **Consistency and escalation:** Have you noticed an increase in the frequency or intensity of this new behavior or substance use? Do you feel the need to hide this behavior or substance use from others?

2. **Reflection and analysis:** After answering the questions, take some time to reflect on your responses. Consider the following questions:

   - Are there any clear patterns or behaviors that indicate you might be substituting one addiction for another?

   - What emotions or triggers are driving these new behaviors or substance use?

   - How is this impacting your overall recovery and well-being?

3. **Action plan:** Based on your reflections, create an action plan to address any potential cross-addictions:

   - **Seek professional help.** Discuss your findings with a therapist or counselor and develop strategies to address underlying issues.

   - **Join support groups.** Participate in support groups that focus on both your initial addiction and any new compulsive behaviors.

   - **Develop healthy coping mechanisms.** Identify and practice healthy coping strategies to manage stress and emotions, such as exercise, meditation, or creative activities.

   - **Monitor and adjust.** Regularly monitor your behaviors and adjust your recovery plan as needed to ensure you are addressing all aspects of your well-being.

By actively identifying and addressing potential cross-addictions, you can strengthen your recovery journey and cultivate a healthier, more fulfilling lifestyle.

At the core of cross-addiction is the idea that addictive behaviors often stem from underlying issues such as trauma, genetic predisposition, or emotional and mental health disorders. When you address the root causes of your addiction, you are better equipped to recognize the patterns that may lead to new compulsive behaviors. This awareness allows you to implement proactive measures, such as engaging in therapy or joining support groups, to mitigate the risk of developing new addictions.

In addition to addressing the root causes of addiction, a comprehensive recovery plan should include a focus on overall well-being. By taking care of your physical, emotional, and mental health, you create a foundation for sustained recovery. This can involve regular exercise, healthy eating, mindfulness practices, and connecting with supportive communities. Incorporating these practices into your daily life can help you manage stress and reduce the likelihood of turning to new addictive behaviors as a coping mechanism.

Mitigating cross-addiction risks

Cross-addiction is the development of a new addiction after recovering from another. To mitigate this risk, adopt a holistic recovery approach:

>> **Address root causes:** Focus on underlying issues like trauma, genetic predisposition, or mental health disorders through therapy and support groups.

>> **Promote overall well-being:** Incorporate regular exercise, healthy eating, and mindfulness practices to maintain physical, emotional, and mental health.

>> **Foster personal growth:** Set achievable goals, celebrate small victories, and build a strong support network to stay motivated and resilient.

By implementing these strategies, you can reduce the risk of cross-addiction and support long-term sobriety and personal growth.

Embracing Sobriety

Achieving sobriety is more than just putting down the bottle or stepping away from substances; it is a holistic journey toward a healthier and more fulfilling life. In this chapter, you will learn what defines sobriety and recovery, where to seek help, how to view relapse, and the importance of continuous sobriety.

Sobriety extends beyond the mere cessation of alcohol or drug use; it encompasses emotional, mental, and social well-being. Embracing this lifestyle involves committing to a series of mindful choices and practices that support overall health and personal growth.

Mindful lifestyle choices

Sobriety is as much about what you do as what you avoid. Nourish your body with nutritious foods, get adequate sleep, and engage in regular physical activity. These practices may seem basic, but they are foundational to building resilience against triggers and stressors.

>> **Mental and emotional health:** Recovery isn't just about stopping substance use; it involves continuous personal growth and addressing the root causes of addiction. This may include therapy to work through trauma, genetic predispositions, or mental health disorders.

>> **Personalized recovery plan:** This is your life, and it's unique to you. Explore what brings you joy and fulfillment, and find ways to integrate these elements into your daily life. This personalized approach can include hobbies, interests, and activities that promote well-being.

>> **Building a support network:** Surround yourself with supportive individuals, whether through peer support groups, family, or friends who understand and respect your sobriety journey. Open communication about your plans and boundaries is crucial for maintaining a safe and supportive environment.

>> **Continuous learning and growth:** Sobriety is a continuous process of self-reflection and growth. Set realistic goals,

celebrate small victories, and remain open to learning new ways to improve your emotional and mental health.

>> **Gratitude and mindfulness practices:** Incorporating mindfulness and gratitude into your daily routine can significantly enhance your recovery journey. These practices help you stay present, appreciate small moments of joy, and build emotional resilience.

By understanding that sobriety is a multifaceted experience, you can appreciate the complexities involved in overcoming addiction. Embrace this comprehensive approach to your journey, focusing on whole-body wellness and personal growth to support long-term sobriety and a fulfilling life.

Sobriety versus recovery

Sobriety is defined as living without alcohol or drugs, encompassing both physical abstinence and a commitment to personal growth. It is not merely about quitting substances; it is about making a conscious and proactive choice to live a life devoid of substances that cause harm. Embracing sobriety means prioritizing your health, both physically and mentally, and understanding that this journey is more than just refraining from using substances. It is about committing to a lifestyle that supports your well-being and fosters positive and lasting changes in your life.

Conversely, recovery extends beyond mere physical cessation and focuses on emotional, mental, and social well-being. While sobriety might be the first step, recovery is the journey that follows, involving *continuous* personal growth and self-awareness. Recovery means uncovering the root causes of addiction, such as trauma or underlying mental health conditions, and seeking to understand the *sparks* and behaviors that led to substance use in the first place. It involves making changes in your life that support your overall health and well-being, whether through therapy, support groups, or other forms of self-care.

Recovery is an ongoing process that demands dedication and effort. It is about more than just stopping the use of substances; it is about creating a new way of living that promotes overall wellness. This journey involves not just the individual but often includes support from friends, family, and professionals who help you navigate the challenges and celebrate the successes. Continuous personal growth is a key component of recovery as you work to build a healthier and more fulfilling life, one day at a time.

REMEMBER

Sobriety is living without alcohol or drugs, focusing on physical abstinence and personal growth, and making conscious choices that prioritize your well-being. Recovery extends beyond just stopping substance use; it involves an ongoing process of emotional, mental, and social well-being. This journey includes continuous personal growth, addressing the root causes of addiction, and making lifestyle changes that support overall health, with dedication and support from friends, family, and professionals.

Where you can get help

Navigating your path to sobriety doesn't have to be a solo endeavor. Various resources can aid in your journey, including rehabilitation centers, support groups, counseling, and hotlines. These resources provide a support system to guide you through the challenges and triumphs of recovery, helping you build resilience and maintain your sobriety.

Rehabilitation centers offer a structured and supportive environment where you can detoxify and receive medical support if necessary. These centers often provide a range of therapies, such as cognitive-behavioral therapy (CBT) and holistic approaches, to address the mental and emotional aspects of addiction. By immersing yourself in a rehabilitation center, you gain access to professionals who can tailor recovery plans to your needs, giving you a solid foundation for long-term sobriety.

Support groups such as Alcoholics Anonymous (AA), SMART (Self-Management and Recovery Training) Recovery, She Recovers, Wellbriety, Narcotics Anonymous (NA), The Buddhist Recovery, and others help create a community of individuals who share similar struggles and goals. These groups provide a platform for sharing experiences, offering mutual encouragement, and learning from others who have successfully navigated their path to recovery. Counseling and therapy play a crucial role in addressing underlying issues that may have contributed to your addiction. You can explore your emotions, develop coping strategies, and work toward long-lasting change through one-on-one sessions with trained mental health professionals. Hotlines offer immediate support and guidance during moments of crisis, ensuring that you're never truly alone in your journey.

TIP

Navigating your path to sobriety doesn't have to be a solo endeavor. Utilize rehabilitation centers for structured environments and tailored recovery plans, support groups like AA or SMART Recovery for community and mutual encouragement, and counseling for addressing underlying issues. These resources collectively help build resilience and maintain your sobriety, offering you a robust support system through the challenges and triumphs of recovery.

Relapse and recovery

Relapse does not have to be a part of your journey, though it can be used as part of your recovery process rather than a failure. It can offer an opportunity to refine coping strategies, understand your sparks, and recommit to your recovery goals. Recognizing that relapse behaviors often manifest before the actual relapse occurs can empower you to address these signs early and adjust your strategies accordingly. Put another way, the drink, or addictive behavior, is the last step in a relapse.

Understanding relapse as part of your journey toward sobriety can fundamentally change how you perceive setbacks. Instead of seeing a relapse as a failure, viewing it as an essential learning experience is more constructive. When you relapse, it provides a window into the aspects of your recovery plan that may need readjustment. For instance, you might discover certain triggers you hadn't previously identified or gaps in your coping mechanisms that need attention. This awareness allows you to tweak your strategies and strengthen your commitment to long-term sobriety.

Additionally, being vigilant about relapse behaviors, which often surface before an actual relapse, equips you with preventive tools. Behaviors such as withdrawing from support groups, neglecting self-care, or romanticizing past substance use are often early indicators. By recognizing these signs, you can pro-actively address the underlying issues before they escalate into a full relapse. Doing so not only helps in maintaining your sobriety but also fosters a deeper understanding of your own triggers and vulnerabilities. This proactive approach makes your path to recovery more resilient and empowers you to make continuous positive changes.

WARNING

Be proactive about relapse. It doesn't have to be part of your journey, but if it occurs, use it as a learning opportunity, not a failure. Understanding that relapse behaviors manifest before the actual relapse can empower you to address these signs early. Behaviors like withdrawing from support groups, neglecting self-care, or romanticizing past substance use are early indicators.

Continuous sobriety

Continuous sobriety involves the ongoing process of maintaining abstinence from alcohol and/ or drugs over a sustained period without relapsing. This commitment goes beyond merely avoiding substances; it encompasses a holistic approach to recovery that reflects an ongoing dedication to a healthier, more fulfilling lifestyle. By choosing continuous sobriety, you are not only saying '"no" to substances but also saying '"yes" to opportunities for personal growth and improved well-being in multiple facets of your life, such as emotional, mental, and social health.

This journey of continuous recovery is a testament to your resilience and determination. Each day presents a new opportunity to evolve and grow, not just in your relationship with substances but in every aspect of your life. Sobriety is not a static goal but a dynamic, lifelong journey that requires you to consistently make choices that align with your values and long-term aspirations. By embracing this path, you commit to improving yourself continuously, understanding that personal growth is an ongoing process, and each small step contributes to your overall journey of recovery and self-improvement.

REMEMBER

Continuous sobriety is not just about avoiding substances; it's an ongoing commitment to a healthier, more fulfilling lifestyle — a healthier you! You create daily choices that support your emotional, mental, and social well-being. Recovery is a dynamic, lifelong process. Each step you take contributes to a better, more fulfilling future.

Chapter **2**

Deciding to Embark on the Sobriety Journey

L iving your life without alcohol can be a courageous and reflective step toward numerous benefits that include healthier relationships, clearer thinking, and overall wellness. This chapter is your practical guide, providing support and direction as you progress toward a healthier, happier life.

Research unequivocally indicates that stepping away from alcohol can lead to profound improvements in sleep quality, immune function, and nutritional health. Without alcohol's sleep disruption, people often experience a more restful and restorative sleep cycle. Moreover, the immune system benefits from the absence of alcohol's suppressive effects, becoming more adept at warding off infections. Lastly, because alcohol is no longer a substitute for nutritious foods, people tend to make healthier dietary choices, improving nutrient absorption and overall well-being. Together, these enhancements contribute to a stronger foundation for a healthier lifestyle.

In this chapter, you will start by examining the need for change, recognizing how alcohol has affected your life, and accepting that a better future starts with embracing change.

Recognizing the Need for Change

Recognizing the need for change is a powerful and challenging step on the path of sobriety. It requires a profound level of honesty with oneself, which can feel as raw as an exposed nerve but is essential. It's the cornerstone on which the long and rewarding journey to recovery is built. Do you suspect, deep down, that you have a problem with alcohol? That nagging doubt — the quiet voice inside whispering that something isn't right — is the seed of awareness you need to nurture.

The journey of sobriety indeed begins with a pivotal moment of self-awareness. It's like that first ray of sunlight piercing through the dark clouds of a stormy horizon, signaling the possibility of a clear sky ahead. You might be feeling the weight of the world right now, but by admitting a need for change, you're taking the most crucial step. This chapter isn't just about guiding you — it's about empowering you to stride through the stubborn fog of denial and emerge into the clarity of truth, where real, profound transformation can begin.

RECLAIMING YOUR LIFE WITH MAI

Mai sat quietly in the dim glow of the morning sun, her coffee cold and untouched. The sounds of the city awakening were muffled by the thick glass of her apartment window. She felt it in this stillness — the undeniable truth that she had been skirting around for years. *She had a problem with alcohol.*

Much like her apartment, Mai's life was neatly organized — a façade of control. But behind closed doors, the recycling bin rattled with the sound of empty bottles, a testament to her nightly battles. The evening ritual had become her secret shame, yet last night had been different. For the first time, she had caught a glimpse of herself in the mirror, the reflection revealing a stranger — a woman who looked tired, defeated, and lost.

In that moment of raw honesty, she realized her life was at a crossroads. The inner voice she had been silencing was now speaking with the force of a tempest, urging her to recognize the need for change. The clarity that washed over her was both terrifying and liberating — terrifying because she knew the road ahead would be riddled with challenges and liberating because she felt an ember of hope ignite within her, something she hadn't felt in years.

Today, Mai would take the first step toward sobriety, the first stride out of the fog. Her hands trembled as she picked up the phone and dialed the number for a local support group. The call was brief, but a weight lifted off her shoulders when she hung up. She had an appointment with a counselor the next day.

As the weeks turned into months, Mai's journey unfolded with determination and grit. Sobriety didn't come easy. There were moments of doubt, cravings, and old habits knocking at her door, but each time, she faced them with the support of her newfound community. Meetings became anchors in her week, and the faces around her, once strangers, turned into mirrors of encouragement.

Mai discovered that in sobriety, she wasn't just abstaining from alcohol; she was reclaiming her life. New friendships blossomed, ones that were authentic and deep. Laughter filled her evenings, and she found joy in the simplicity of life's little moments — joy that no drink could ever provide.

Years later, Mai would often share her story, speaking hope into the hearts of those curious about becoming sober. She was straight to the point because she knew lives were on the line. She would tell them about her first step, about the morning when the clarity of truth shone through her window, offering a promise of a life she could have never dreamed of — a life filled with community, laughter, and good people — a life truly lived.

Acknowledging the impact of substance use

The realization of substance use impact is a profound awakening. It demands honesty and courage to see and accept how alcohol or drugs have affected your health, finances, relationships, and overall life trajectory. This process of acknowledgment isn't a quest to dwell on the past; instead, it's an act of bravery to face the reality of one's condition. It's about understanding that the side effects of substance use are not badges of honor or symbols of a life well-lived but signs that point to a more profound *unease*, a malfunction that must not be ignored. It takes immense strength to hold oneself accountable for the damage done to oneself and the people and communities around us.

REMEMBER

This moment of reckoning is not about assigning blame but taking responsibility. It comes with accepting that one's behavior is neither sustainable nor conducive to genuine happiness or purpose. By recognizing the link between substance use and the diminishing joy in your life, you'll ignite the flames of motivation needed to fuel your journey toward sobriety.

Asking yourself how substance use has affected you

As you embark on your sobriety journey, it's essential to take a moment for self-reflection. To help you assess the impact of substance use on your life, consider the following questions:

>> Has my substance use negatively impacted my physical or mental health?

>> Has my financial stability ever suffered because of my alcohol or drug use?

>> Have my relationships with others been damaged due to my substance use habits?

>> Has my substance use caused me to stray from my goals and passions in life?

>> Am I avoiding the truth about the sustainability of my behavior and the responsibility for its effects on myself and others?

TIP

While these yes or no questions can be starting points for reflection, remember that the complexities of substance use and its impact are rarely black and white. It might be beneficial to follow up any "yes" with a more detailed exploration to fully understand the scope and nuances of the issue at hand.

For example, if you answered "yes" to the third question about substance use affecting your relationships, take a moment to explore this further.

Think about a relationship that has been strained or broken due to your habits. Was it a close friendship that started to fade because you missed important events or appeared distant? Or was it a romantic partnership that suffered due to your unpredictable behavior or lack of presence? Reflect on the emotions this evokes, both in yourself and in the other person.

Assess how your substance use contributed to the issues and consider what changes could be made to heal or improve these relationships. Acknowledging these feelings and consequences is important, as they can be powerful motivators for change and provide a clearer picture of the paths to mend and nurture your connections with others.

For example, you might consider your past friendship(s) with an old college roommate(s) that deteriorated as your drinking escalated. You used to share laughs and support each other's ambitions, but over time, you began to cancel plans last minute or show up intoxicated. This behavior left your friend feeling disregarded and hurt, leading to a rift between you.

As you recall the sense of loss and the guilt that accompanies it, understand how your substance use played a role in this falling out. Envision the steps you can take to rebuild trust and camaraderie, such as reaching out to catch up, perhaps apologizing for that old behavior, and then making it a point to be present at future gatherings or simply listening. Acknowledging the damage done and your part in it can be a poignant incentive for recovery and restoring the bonds you once cherished.

Walking through consequences

Consequences manifest their roots in every corner of life disturbed by substance abuse. Financial woes, such as bankruptcy, can be a wake-up call, crystalizing the long-term cost of addiction. The pain of personal loss — whether losing loved ones or the stark realization that one's potential is slipping away — can serve as a powerful wake-up call. The fabric of life, woven with plans and aspirations, may start to unravel. Career setbacks, health issues, and diminishing self-esteem often follow a path paved by substance dependency. Each car accident, each hospital visit, and every estranged family member is a waypoint on a map that leads toward an inevitable conclusion: *change is not merely a choice; it's a necessity.*

In facing these consequences, there's an opportunity to assess the damage done and to decide what matters most. Being honest about how alcohol or drugs have steered you off course isn't a weakness — it's the groundwork for building a courageous, more fulfilling life. This reflection is a pivotal starting point for those deciding to embark on the sobriety journey. Take inventory of the consequences you've encountered, and let them motivate you to pursue a path where your actions align with your values and hopes. Each sober day becomes a step away from the fallout of the past toward a horizon of regained purpose and joy.

The Mindset for Sobriety

Embarking on the sobriety journey is not merely a lifestyle change; it's a profound transformation of the mind. It's about restructuring our thoughts and attitudes toward life's challenges and our means of confronting them. To become sober and thrive in that sobriety, one must adopt a mindset that fosters growth, resilience, and self-compassion. In this section, you will explore how you can cultivate such a mindset and open the doors to a more purposeful and joyous existence.

Creating and cultivating a growth mindset

At the heart of any sobriety journey lies the choice to grow — to evolve beyond our current selves and the patterns that bind us. This concept of a growth mindset is the belief that our essential qualities are things we can cultivate through our efforts. Where once you saw a dead end, with a growth mindset, you learned to see a path forward.

The realization may come in waves of desperation or quiet moments of reflection: the understanding that your lifestyle is unsustainable. This is often the first step, recognizing the need for change. But where do we go from there? The answer is simple yet challenging — we must embrace the unknown and be willing to learn from each misstep along the way.

Start acknowledging the need to change and understand that mistakes are not a reflection of your worth but learning opportunities. Shift the focus from what you are losing (alcohol) to what you're gaining — an enhanced understanding of yourself, improved health, stronger relationships, and reclaimed control over your finances and decisions.

Developing a growth mindset is critical for embracing sobriety and can be cultivated through these five practical steps:

1. **Embrace learning over perfection:** Understand that sobriety is a learning process, not a destination, where everything immediately becomes perfect. Accept failures and setbacks as opportunities for growth and learning. Every mistake can be a step forward because you gain insight that you didn't have before.

2. **Celebrate small victories:** In your journey, it's crucial to recognize and celebrate your progress, no matter how small. Each day of sobriety, every challenge overcome, and each time you say no to temptation are significant milestones. These small victories accumulate and lead to lasting transformation.

3. **Seek feedback and support:** Open yourself up to feedback from trusted friends, mentors, or support groups. Growth happens in community and dialogue. Being receptive to the experiences and advice of others can provide new perspectives and encourage persistence in your journey.

4. **Cultivate self-compassion:** Be kind to yourself. Understand that self-criticism and harsh self-judgment are counterproductive. Practice self-compassion by speaking to yourself with the same kindness and understanding that you would offer a good friend.

5. **Set flexible goals:** Establish clear, achievable goals with the willingness to adapt as needed. Your path to sobriety may have unexpected turns, so maintaining flexibility in your goals can help you stay committed without becoming discouraged by rigid expectations.

REMEMBER

Adopting a growth mindset is a daily practice. You need to work on it, continuously reinforcing these steps; this way of thinking will become second nature over time. As you progress, you will notice improvements in your sobriety and all areas of your life, leading to a more purposeful and joyous existence. Stay confident and committed to your growth, and the results will follow.

Focusing on self-compassion and resilience — but never just one

Walking down the road of sobriety, you will encounter hurdles that test your resolve. Self-compassion and resilience must become your closest allies to overcome these and thrive. They are two sides of the same coin, essential and complementary.

Self-compassion involves recognizing that suffering and personal inadequacy are part of the shared human experience. You are not alone, and it's okay not to be okay. You offer kindness and understanding instead of mercilessly judging yourself for any shortcomings. Resilience is your capacity to rebound from adversity, building strength through your experiences.

Resilience is bolstered in the company of a supportive community that can lend strength and share the burden of tough situations. It grows not from toughing it out alone but from the collective wisdom and support that come when you bravely reach out and express vulnerability.

REMEMBER

You need both self-compassion and resilience in the face of these barriers to guide you through moments of doubt and to remind you of your worth and strength. Together, they weave a safety net of mental well-being, nurturing you as you learn, falter, and ultimately soar on your journey to sobriety.

Breaking Down Barriers to Sobriety

Embarking on a sobriety journey is akin to setting sail into the vast, open waters of the unknown; it's a voyage that demands courage, determination, and an unyielding spirit. To navigate these waters, you must break down barriers that have long held you in the grip of dependency, each one a blockade to the serene harbor of sober living. Explore these barriers and chart a course through them by identifying your triggers and releasing yourself from the chains of stigma.

Identifying and addressing your triggers

Our daily lives are intricately woven with patterns and influences that nudge us toward old habits, the siren call of alcohol. These triggers can be as overt as a social event where drinks are flowing freely or as subtle as an emotional state of stress or boredom. Recognizing these triggers is the first act of reclaiming power over your choices.

REMEMBER

The journey begins with honest self-reflection. Delve into your routines, relationships, and emotional states to unearth the signals that precede the desire for a drink. Once identified, construct new, healthier rituals. Replace the after-work beer with a jog in the park or the weekend binge with a creative hobby. The goal is to rewire our responses to these triggers, creating new neural pathways that favor sobriety over intoxication.

Moreover, you should not embark upon this phase alone — seeking the support of professionals, counselors, and support groups can provide the guidance and affirmation needed to move forward. Equipped with scientific knowledge about the nature of addiction, you empower yourself further, understanding that this is not a matter of sheer willpower but rather a complex interplay of biology and the environment.

In addressing triggers, it's crucial to foster a mindset of resilience and self-compassion. There will be challenging moments, but these challenges will strengthen your resolve. As you practice self-compassion, you become more forgiving of your missteps, understanding that each one is a lesson rather than a failure.

TIP

Creating new habits to diminish the power of triggers is a fundamental step toward achieving long-term sobriety. Here are three practical steps:

>> **Conduct a trigger audit:** Write down the triggers that provoke your desire to drink. Be honest and thorough. Include specific scenarios, emotional states, people, and even times of day. This self-awareness is a powerful tool in changing your behavioral responses.

>> **Design healthier alternatives:** For every trigger you identify, craft a positive habit to counter it. If stress tempts you to drink, plan a relaxation routine like meditation or a warm bath. Replace the after-work drink with exercise or a new hobby that engages and fulfills you.

>> **Cultivate resilience and practice self-compassion:** Prepare mentally for the reality that the path will have its difficulties. Treat yourself with the same kindness you would offer a friend when you encounter them. Remember, every challenge is an opportunity to strengthen your commitment to sobriety.

By diligently implementing these steps, you will start redirecting your reactions to triggers, forming new, healthier neural pathways. The key is consistency and the willingness to persist, even when it's tough. Be patient, and trust that each step you take builds a more resilient, sober you.

Overcoming stigma

One of the most insidious obstacles faced on the road to recovery is the stigma attached to alcoholism. Societal misconceptions paint a picture of the person struggling with alcohol as someone who lacks self-discipline or moral fiber. It is crucial to destroy these fallacies, building instead a narrative of sobriety that honors the strength and courage needed to step away from alcohol.

TIP

To dismantle this stigma, you must start by speaking openly about your battles with addiction, sharing your stories with both vulnerability and valor. In doing so, you lay bare the truth that alcoholism is not a weakness but a health challenge that many face.

Community and connection play pivotal roles in overcoming stigma. Surround yourself with those who understand your plight and can offer empathy and evidence of a life beyond addiction. Integrate into movements and groups where sobriety is not only normalized but celebrated.

Finally, advocate for a change in the societal portrayal of drinking. Challenge media depictions that glamorize alcohol and expose the harsh realities of its grip. We can begin to tear down the walls of judgment and shame by facing these truths head-on and with the collective might of a supportive community.

REMEMBER

The decision to pursue sobriety isn't just a personal milestone; it's a societal transformation. As we work individually to find our purpose and joy beyond the veil of alcohol, collectively, we craft a new, sober reality — one filled with authenticity, health, and boundless joy.

FROM CONCEALMENT TO COURAGE WITH JAMES

In the throes of addiction, James was a man haunted by the incessant need for alcohol. His life had become a series of carefully orchestrated maneuvers to conceal his drinking: the clinking bottles hidden in the shadows of his closet, the lies to cover up the pervasive scent of liquor on his breath, and the excuses for why he was perpetually late for work. His world was a blur in which the lines — literally and metaphorically — were increasingly hard to keep straight. He drove under the influence, a dangerous gamble he made all too often, and he found himself sipping from a flask at his son's games.

But amidst the chaos, a moment of clarity pierced through the fog: the realization that he could not go on like this. With a heavy heart, James sought help. The tools of recovery became his lifeline: meetings where confessions and life lessons intermingled, therapy sessions began to untangle the knots of his psyche, and unwavering support of friends who had once been strangers in similar struggles.

As James reconstructed his life, he noticed the societal stigma that clung to his past self — the sideways glances when he turned down a drink, the whispers of *"alcoholic"* that felt like brands on his skin. These misconceptions equated his disease with a lack of self-control. James took a stand and was no longer a prisoner of these falsehoods. He openly shared his journey, speaking at community centers and schools, bringing humanity to the statistic of alcoholism.

He described the realities of addiction and how it had strained his relationships, jeopardized his job, and compromised his role as a parent. He also spoke of the monumental strength it took to break free, stand tall amidst the wreckage, and choose a different path. James became an active member of movements that celebrated sobriety.

James's advocacy extended to challenging the media's glamorization of drinking, emphasizing the need for more honest representations that acknowledged the pain and the struggle, as well as the possibility of redemption. His message was clear: Recovering from alcoholism was not a solitary triumph but a collective victory for society, a step toward a future where authenticity and health were at the forefront.

Through consistent effort and the collective might of a supportive community, James helped to dismantle the walls of judgment and shame. His story became a beacon of hope, illuminating the truth that overcoming alcoholism is not a question of morality but a courageous battle against a formidable health challenge.

The societal stigma that had once seemed impenetrable began to dissipate. In its place grew a new understanding — one that recognized the bravery of those like James who fought to reclaim their lives. His transformation was more than personal; it was a testament to the societal change that occurs when we view sobriety as a personal milestone and a redefinition of strength and resilience.

James's life, once ruled by the need to hide, was now an open book — a narrative that inspired others and shifted the societal perspective. He stood as living proof that in sobriety, there is not only recovery but also the potential to rewrite the script of one's life, to emerge from the stigma, and into a reality filled with boundless joy and unshakeable authenticity.

REMEMBER

This chapter introduced you to the significant yet rewarding journey toward long-term sobriety. It requires bravery, introspection, and a genuine resolve for transformation. Sobriety redefines your self-relationship and interactions with others, bringing mental clarity, better health, and genuine relationships. You'll find evidence-based knowledge and narratives, illustrating the impact of your decision to begin and deepen your recovery process. This chapter highlights the importance of recognizing the role of substance use in your life as a foundation for change. It guides you in developing a mindset focused on growth and resilience, which is essential for handling challenges and confronting stigma. Remember that sobriety is not about what you give up; rather, it's about the valuable gains in health, joy, and self-discovery.

Chapter **3**

Overcoming Emotional Challenges in Your Recovery

E mbracing the full spectrum of your emotions is integral to navigating the journey through long-term sobriety. When you first step into this new phase of life, it can be as though you're emerging from a prolonged stay in darkness into an intense luminosity that exposes every hidden corner of your being. This light of sobriety reveals the full array of feelings you may have previously dimmed with alcohol or addictive behaviors, presenting both challenges and an opportunity for profound personal growth. Living emotionally sober means facing these sometimes overwhelming feelings head-on, allowing for an internal transformation that is as enriching as it is essential.

In this chapter, you'll take a closer look at how to manage your emotions constructively, highlighting the importance of developing coping mechanisms for a stable and fulfilling sober life. You'll explore strategies ranging from mindfulness techniques to cultivating a supportive community. Such tools are not just about fending off your discomfort with raw, unfiltered emotions but about learning to thrive in their presence. With each step forward, the once-blinding light begins to soften, revealing a path of self-discovery full of joy and insights only accessible through the clarity of a sober mind.

Understanding The Power of Your Emotions

Navigating long-term sobriety requires a keen understanding of how emotions can shape your experiences. Scientific research supports the theory that emotions play a vital role in decision-making, influencing behavior and well-being. In sobriety, this becomes particularly pronounced. Studies have shown that emotional regulation improves with sustained abstinence, enhancing one's ability to cope with stressors and reducing the likelihood of relapse. Moreover, neuroscientific findings indicate that the brain's neuroplasticity allows for rewiring reward pathways, leading to healthier emotional responses over time. Embracing and understanding the power of your emotions in long-term sobriety is not just anecdotal; it is supported by empirical evidence that underscores the transformative potential of living sober.

REMEMBER

As time passes in your journey of long-term sobriety, the room that once felt overwhelmingly bright begins to feel more familiar. The blinding intensity gradually softens into a warm glow, gently illuminating your path of self-discovery and future growth. Living in sustained abstinence means becoming attuned to the ebb and flow of your emotions without the need for numbing agents or behaviors. It means embracing the full range of feelings — joy, sadness, uncertainty, anger, and everything in between — as integral parts of your human experience. Sober life is about embracing the light and shadows within yourself and finding harmony in the beautiful complexity of your emotional landscape.

Here, you'll identify personal downfalls, a transformative journey that paves your path to an empowered, sober life. Through raw and revealing narratives, you'll learn that facing the emotional realities of early sobriety is not a regression but a courageous step toward genuine growth and healing.

Identifying personal downfalls

Realizing where you stumble is the first step in regaining your footing. Many in early sobriety feel emotionally juvenile — as if reverting to their teenage years, with a surge of feelings they thought they had outgrown. This sensation is not regression; it is an awakening to the emotional growth that was stunted when you sought support from alcohol.

It's vital to inventory your emotional responses during this period. Acknowledge how you might deflect, withdraw, or lash out when uncomfortable. Sobriety demands that you face yourself — to confront your tendencies, all of them, head-on. You must ask what personal downfalls manifest as defensiveness or evasion. These are hard questions. As uncomfortable as it is, identifying these downfalls isn't self-deprecation but an act of courage — it is choosing to own our story fully.

TIP

Identifying your downfalls involves answering key questions regarding self-awareness, such as recognizing the specific emotions you feel when uncomfortable and how they manifest in your behavior; reflecting on defense mechanisms by analyzing situations where you deflect, withdraw, or lash out and understanding the reasons behind these actions; conducting an honest self-assessment to pinpoint tendencies of defensiveness or evasion and their spark. Understanding how you typically react to sparks and how you can respond more constructively in the future.

Identify personal downfalls by answering these questions:

>> **Self-awareness:** What specific emotions do I feel when I'm uncomfortable, and how do they usually manifest in my behavior?

>> **Reflection on defense mechanisms:** In which situations am I most likely to deflect, withdraw, or lash out, and why might that be?

>> **Honest self-assessment:** What are my personal tendencies that can be seen as defensiveness or evasion, and what triggers these responses?

>> **Understanding triggers:** When I encounter a trigger, how do I typically react, and how can I respond more constructively in the future?

>> **Recognizing patterns:** Are there any recurring patterns in my behavior that undermine my sobriety, and how can I address them effectively?

>> **Personal downfalls:** What personal downfalls contribute to my defensiveness, and how can I work on accepting and improving these areas?

>> **Coping strategies:** What healthy coping strategies can I implement to deal with discomfort without resorting to old habits?

>> **Embracing vulnerability:** How can I become more comfortable feeling vulnerable as a part of my journey toward owning my story?

>> **Ownership of actions:** How can I take greater responsibility for my actions and reactions, even when it's challenging to do so?

>> **Commitment to growth:** How can I reaffirm my commitment to personal growth and sobriety daily, especially when faced with adversity?

IDENTIFYING HIS ACTIONS WITH LAWRENCE

Lawrence was driven by an unquenchable thirst for success in his career. He clocked countless late hours at the office, constantly pushing for the next achievement, the next award — but at a price. His obsession with work meant deadlines took precedence over everything else, including the mundane task of submitting expense reports. This oversight led to delays in his payments, brewing a storm at home.

Equally stressed about their financial well-being, his wife would confront Lawrence, her worry manifesting regret and anger. Never equipped with the tools to deal with confrontation healthily, Lawrence escaped through the bottle and sports betting. With his mind perpetually distracted, he would miss deadlines and instigate more arguments, and the cycle seemed never to end.

Drinking became his method of deflection, an escape from facing the issues that so desperately needed his attention.

Realizing where you stumble is the first step in regaining your footing.

Late one evening, Lawrence sat in his dimly lit living room, the television flickering shadows as yet another game unfolded before an audience of one. At this moment, amidst the noise of the crowd from the TV, Lawrence heard something else — the sound of his inner turmoil.

For the first time in years, Lawrence felt the full weight of his emotional stunting. It was as if he had suddenly awakened from a long, intoxicating slumber.

Early sobriety demands you to face yourself and confront your tendencies head-on.

That night, Lawrence chose the solitude of his living room. It was not about stopping drinking; it was about starting to live. He acknowledged his downfalls, to no longer deflect or withdraw from the life

(continued)

(continued)

he was responsible for. A daunting task lay ahead, but Lawrence knew he needed to own the story that was his to tell.

The following day, Lawrence reached out for support. He joined a sobriety group, individuals who knew the struggle of confronting their demons. Together, they would share their vulnerabilities and triumphs. Through this community, he learned the value of authentic friendships — those created under the recognition of mutual struggle and perseverance.

In the following weeks and months, Lawrence worked to unravel the habits that had led to the isolation and debt. He set a strict schedule, asked for some time off work, and communicated openly with his wife. That month, his expense reports were turned in on time, and the chaos at home began to subside. More importantly, he learned to find joy outside the office and the nightly sporting game or event! He finally said yes to his wife's request to go to a nonsporting event, and he began to discover hobbies that engaged his mind without needing a drink in his hand.

As uncomfortable as it is, identifying these downfalls isn't self-deprecation but an act of courage.

Lawrence's story is one of resilience. He faced his vulnerabilities head-on, learning that acknowledging his downfalls was not an act of self-deprecation but of courage. Lawrence now understood that his greatest strength was not in the solitary pursuit of professional success but in the shared journey toward emotional maturity and inner peace. His peace of mind became his priority.

The reality of the struggle is about facing the hard truths, embracing the discomfort, and finding a path through it. Sobriety isn't just about removing alcohol — it's about gaining a life beyond anything you could have once imagined for yourself.

Exploring resentments

Resentments in recovery are like weights that anchor you to your past, hindering your ability to move freely into a fulfilling future. To explore these resentments is to dive deeply into your psyche, uncovering the root causes of anger and bitterness. An essential part of this journey is recognizing these resentments openly and impartially.

Bringing your resentments into the open is the first critical step toward resolving them. This process often involves clear and honest communication with those involved, but the most transformative aspect is the act of forgiveness. Forgiving oneself and others is a powerful step that shouldn't be misinterpreted as a sign of weakness; rather, it is a profound statement of inner power. Forgiveness demonstrates the courage to acknowledge mistakes and grievances while choosing to break free from their hold on you.

Forgiveness denotes a commitment to moving beyond the entanglements of past conflicts, nurturing a mindset that encourages personal growth and emotional healing. When you forgive, you're not just releasing others from the blame but liberating yourself from the cycle of negative emotions that can impede your progress. It's an active endeavor to rebuild your well-being on a foundation of understanding and compassion. This process not only cultivates a more resilient spirit but also paves the way toward rebuilding trust and restoring relationships. Forgiveness is the cornerstone of meaningful change, allowing you to transform pain into purpose and conflict into peace. It creates the possibility for new beginnings and the opportunity to experience life unburdened by the weight of unresolved emotions.

It's important to note that unresolved resentments can lead to emotional turmoil and, in some cases, relapse. Understanding the impact of resentment on your sobriety journey is crucial. For further insights on preventing relapse, you can explore the topic in more detail in Chapter 10, where we further discuss the complexities surrounding relapse and the role of emotional triggers in recovery. Resolving resentments is a key aspect of maintaining emotional sobriety and adaptability on the path to lasting recovery.

Mapping emotional responses

Every emotion has a corresponding action or reaction. As you commit to a journey of sustained abstinence, it is imperative to uncover the origins of your emotional responses. These responses serve as your intrinsic guidance system, and fully comprehending them equates to possessing a nautical chart for your inner psychological terrain.

Your goal is to cultivate a *self-check-in* procedure when emotional turbulence hits. This process involves crafting a mental sanctuary where you can take a moment, inhale deeply, and evaluate the true nature of your inner experiences. Rather than being overwhelmed by a surge of emotions, you master the art of riding them, gracefully navigating the currents until you find yourself in a state of tranquility.

TIP

You can build an arsenal of coping strategies — whether writing down thoughts, engaging in physical activity, or seeking connection through conversation. These skills bolster your emotional resilience, allowing you to remain connected with yourself and your emotions without being driven by them. As you learn to understand the power of your feelings, you unlock a new dimension of sobriety — as emotionally enriching as liberating.

Charting emotions and responses in sobriety

It's essential to see and recognize the contrast when living sober, as the differences between life with substance use and life in sobriety are profound and often transformative. Take, for example, the change in how you interact with daily routines and responsibilities. When in the grip of addiction, even simple tasks may have felt overwhelming, shrouded in a fog of lethargy or disinterest; paying your bills on time, managing the household, and even caring for family members can be too much. In sobriety, there's often a renewed energy and focus, allowing for a re-engagement with work, hobbies, and self-care that were once neglected.

Even your sensory clarity emerges. Where once the flavors of a meal might have been dulled or forgotten, sobriety allows you to savor each bite, appreciate the textures, and delight in the aromas. Social interactions, too, shift dramatically. Instead of forging connections through a shared haze of intoxication, sober relationships are built on genuine understanding and mutual support. Discussions are remembered, bonds are strengthened, and trust is rebuilt.

Sobriety reveals your emotional contrasts within oneself. Before, emotions may have been muted or masked by substance use; now, they can cascade with intensity. Joy may feel more vivid, sorrow may carry a new depth, and anger may demand constructive outlets. Navigating this emotional landscape can be challenging, yet it's also an opportunity for growth. Learning to experience and process emotions without the veil of substances leads to a richer, more authentic life.

Recognizing these contrasts is about seeing and feeling the changes deeply and understanding the full extent of sobriety's impact. It's a realization that life in sobriety is not simply a life without substances; it's a new narrative, rich with potential for rediscovery and reinvention.

Table 3-1 illustrates potential emotional responses without the clarity that sobriety can bring. This chart reflects how emotions might be handled in unhealthy ways, which might occur when you or someone is struggling with substance use or is not practicing sobriety.

TABLE 3-1   **Emotions and Unhealthy Responses Without Sobriety**

Emotion	Unhealthy Response Strategies
Anxiety	• Resort to substance use to numb feelings • Avoid facing the source of anxiety through escapism
Sadness	• Isolate oneself and potentially use substances to temporarily alleviate the pain • Avoid discussing or expressing feelings
Anger	• Respond impulsively with aggression or substance use • Hold onto grudges and resentment without seeking resolution
Frustration	• Give up on tasks or challenges quickly • Engage in self-sabotaging behavior
Loneliness	• Withdraw from social interactions • Rely on substances for a sense of comfort or connection

(continued)

TABLE 3-1 *(continued)*

Emotion	Unhealthy Response Strategies
Happiness	• Use substances to enhance or prolong the feeling of happiness • Fail to recognize and appreciate the moment without external stimuli
Boredom	• Turn to substance use for excitement or stimulation • Lack of motivation to seek out healthy and engaging activities
Overwhelm	• Feel paralyzed and unable to take action • Increase substance use as a coping mechanism for stress
Guilt	• Dwell on past mistakes without seeking resolution or forgiveness • Potentially use substances to escape feelings of guilt
Hopelessness	• Succumb to negative thinking without seeking help • Possibly use substances to cope with despair
Gratitude	• Struggle to feel or express genuine gratitude • Overlook positive aspects of life due to a focus on negative experiences or substance use
Pride	• Fail to acknowledge personal achievements or attribute them to substance use • Possess a distorted view of self-worth

Having this chart as a comparison can serve as a powerful tool in highlighting the benefits of sobriety and the risks associated with substance use. It can also underscore seeking help and adopting healthier coping mechanisms.

Table 3-2 contrasts with Table 3-1, identifying healthy response strategies for living a sober life; these are general suggestions; it's important to note that your responses to emotions will vary.

TABLE 3-2	**Healthy Response Strategies**
Emotion	Healthy Response Strategies
Anxiety	• Practice deep breathing, meditation, or yoga. • Engage in physical exercise. • Talk to a supportive friend or therapist.
Sadness	• Allow yourself to cry and express your feelings. • Write in a journal. Listen to soothing music. • Seek out comforting activities or hobbies.
Anger	• Take a timeout to cool down. • Engage in physical activity to release tension. • Give yourself permission to be angry, but don't hang onto it. • Use conflict resolution skills.
Frustration	• Break tasks into smaller steps. • Take a break and return with a fresh perspective. • Discuss your feelings with someone you trust.
Loneliness	• Reach out to friends or support groups. • Volunteer or join community activities. • Adopt a pet if possible.
Happiness	• Share your joy with others. • Practice gratitude. • Save the moment in a journal or by taking photos.
Boredom	• Explore new hobbies or interests. • Create a routine with varied activities. • Challenge yourself with new goals.
Overwhelm	• Prioritize tasks and delegate when possible. • Say no to additional responsibilities. • Practice self-care.
Guilt	• Make amends if necessary. • Learn from the experience. • Forgive yourself and move forward.

(continued)

CHAPTER 3 **Overcoming Emotional Challenges in Your Recovery**   47

TABLE 3-2 *(continued)*

Emotion	Healthy Response Strategies
Hopelessness	• Set small, achievable goals.
	• Seek professional help if needed.
	• Connect with others who have overcome similar challenges.
Gratitude	• Express thanks to others.
	• Volunteer or give back to the community.
	• Reflect on positive changes in your life.
Pride	• Celebrate your accomplishments.
	• Share your success story to inspire others.
	• Remember the journey that led to this point.

JOURNEY FROM NUMBNESS TO MINDFULNESS IN SOBRIETY WITH JOHN

John struggled with alcohol dependency for several years. When he decided to seek sobriety, he was overwhelmed by the intense emotions that he had been numbing with alcohol. He felt particularly challenged by anxiety and loneliness. However, John found a sobriety workbook with a chart similar to Table 3-2.

He began to practice the healthy response strategies listed above whenever he experienced anxiety — deep breathing exercises became a part of his daily routine; he also joined a local yoga class. When feelings of loneliness crept in, he reached out to a support group specifically for individuals in recovery. John found that sharing his experiences with others who understood his struggle was incredibly comforting.

Over time, John learned to anticipate his emotional imbalances and prepared himself with healthy responses. He learned the importance of surrounding himself with supportive friends and family. When he felt happiness or gratitude, he shared these feelings and recognized them as milestones in his recovery!

REMEMBER

In your quest for sobriety, embracing emotional challenges as opportunities for growth becomes a pivotal part of your journey. Consider this list as your trusty compass, guiding you through the uncharted territories of your inner world. Each suggestion offers a meaningful way to engage with your emotions, craft a supportive environment, and celebrate your progress with tangible actions. Start charting your personalized map to resilience and empowerment, one heartfelt step at a time.

Following are some suggestions for taking on emotional challenges:

>> **Create a personalized emotion journal:** Keep a journal that tracks your emotions and how you respond to them. This can help you become more aware of your patterns and avoid unhealthy coping mechanisms.

>> **Develop a support network:** Build relationships with people who are supportive of your sobriety. This could include friends, family members, or individuals from support groups.

>> **Learn new skills:** Engage in activities such as cooking, art, or playing a musical instrument, filling your time and providing a sense of accomplishment and pride.

>> **Set realistic goals:** Work toward achievable goals that provide direction and purpose. Each goal reached is a testament to your strength in sobriety.

>> **Exercise regularly:** Physical activity is beneficial for health and a natural way to boost mood and reduce stress.

>> **Celebrate sobriety milestones:** Acknowledge your sober time with small celebrations or rewards. This can help maintain motivation and pride in your progress.

REMEMBER

Recovery is a personal journey, and what works for one person may not work for another. Finding the tools and strategies that resonate with you and support your path to sobriety is important.

Developing Coping Mechanisms

In early sobriety, it feels like all the emotions you suppressed with alcohol suddenly flood back in with an intensity that can be hard to manage. You can often feel emotionally underdeveloped as if you're an adolescent just learning to navigate your feelings without the buffer of alcohol. You can overcome these challenges by developing coping mechanisms that support your emotional journey toward a healthier, sober you.

To develop coping mechanisms, you need to understand what emotional regulation is. Emotional regulation refers to the processes by which individuals influence which emotions they experience, when they encounter them, and how they express and feel them. It is an intrinsic and extrinsic mechanism meant to monitor, evaluate, and modulate emotional reactions, whether to dampen, intensify, maintain, or change them.

Effective emotional regulation involves being aware of one's emotional responses and utilizing strategies to manage and cope appropriately. This can include being mindful of the situation and potential triggers, engaging in deep breathing or meditation to reduce arousal, reframing the situation to alter its emotional impact, or seeking support from others to help process emotions.

Emotional regulation is crucial for psychological well-being and social functioning. It allows you to respond to life's challenges flexibly and socially appropriately, contributing to personal and relational stability. Difficulties with emotional regulation can lead to emotional distress and are associated with a variety of mental health disorders, including mood and anxiety disorders, personality disorders, and relapse.

ENGAGING WITH COGNITIVE BEHAVIORAL THERAPY (CBT) SKILLS

Let's say you attend a wedding reception where old friends, unaware of your journey to sobriety, enthusiastically encourage you to toast with champagne. The festive atmosphere and the presence of alcohol at every table make it a challenging scenario, tempting you to join in as you used to do in the past. Following are some ways you could handle the situation:

Cognitive Behavioral Therapy (CBT) is a scientifically validated form of psychotherapy that helps people of all types identify and alter negative thought patterns contributing to emotional distress. CBT aims to transform the emotional responses stemming from those thoughts by challenging and reframing irrational or maladaptive thoughts, leading to more balanced behaviors.

Use CBT techniques to identify thought patterns that suggest one drink won't hurt and counter them with rational responses. This practice, known as cognitive restructuring, teaches you to dispute and replace detrimental thoughts with more balanced, factual representations, aiding in the regulation of your emotional responses and supporting your sobriety journey.

Identifying thought patterns

- **Your strategy:** Use CBT techniques to identify your thought patterns that suggest one drink won't hurt and counter your thoughts with rational responses.

- **Example:** You can take a moment to step away from the crowd, reminding yourself of your progress and how much you've worked to achieve your current state of sobriety. You recognize that "just one drink" can undermine your efforts and instead prepare a polite but firm refusal like, "Thank you, but I'm celebrating in my own way tonight."

(continued)

(continued)

Planning and rehearsing responses

- **Your strategy:** Before attending events where alcohol will be present, plan and rehearse your responses to drink offers.

- **Example:** Anticipating the situation, you already prepared a variety of responses ranging from a simple "No, thanks" to more detailed explanations if pressed, such as, "I've found that I enjoy these special occasions even more when I'm fully present, so I prefer not to drink."

The buddy system

- **Your strategy:** Attend social gatherings with a sober friend or someone aware of your sobriety and can offer support.

- **Example:** You arrange to attend the wedding with a friend who is also sober. You both agree to stick together during the event, providing mutual support and camaraderie when declining drinks. If the pressure becomes too intense, you have an exit strategy plan to leave the event early together, ensuring your sobriety remains intact.

By utilizing these coping strategies, you are better equipped to maintain sobriety in social situations where alcohol is present and pressure to drink may arise. It's important to highlight that while a range of strategies can be effective, their success often depends on the individual's commitment to their recovery and the support systems they have in place.

Building your toolbox of strategies

The journey to sobriety is not just about abstaining from alcohol; it's about rebuilding a life that you can live without needing to escape. A vital part of this process is gathering a set of reliable strategies to cope with the emotional waves without being pulled under. Think of it as creating a personalized toolbox you can always carry. Inside this toolbox, you might place mindfulness techniques — such as meditation or deep-breathing exercises, to calm the mind when stressors arise. Add in physical activity, a proven mood stabilizer, from a brisk walk to a high-intensity workout, whatever works for you.

Include creative outlets like journaling, which is a powerful tool for processing thoughts. Music, art, and other forms of self-expression also provide therapeutic ways to deal with emotions. And let's not forget the power of community. Building strong, understanding relationships creates an environment where you can be open about your feelings and seek support when needed.

Putting this toolbox together in today's busy world can be difficult. Here are some questions that you can use in building your personalized toolbox for sobriety:

Creating mindful moments:

>> What moments in your day could you incorporate brief meditation or mindfulness practices in your day?

>> How do you typically react to stress, and which mindfulness techniques do you find most appealing to counteract that reaction?

Let's get physical:

>> What forms of physical activity do you enjoy, and how can you integrate them into your regular routine?

>> How does your body respond to exercise, and do you notice a difference in your stress levels or mood afterward?

>> Could you set a small, realistic fitness goal to work toward each week?

Creativity outlet:

>> What creative activities do you find fulfilling or have always wanted to try?

>> When do you feel most inspired to create, and how can you make time for that in your schedule?

>> What kind of music uplifts you or helps you relax, and how can you use it as a tool for your sobriety?

>> Are there any art projects or musical endeavors you've put off that you can now use as an outlet for expression?

>> How can engaging with music or art help to distract or soothe you when you're encountering difficult emotions?

Find a new community and relationships:

>> In your life, who can you count on for understanding and support as you work toward sobriety?

>> Can you join support groups or communities to enhance your sense of belonging and shared experience?

>> How can you actively cultivate and strengthen these relationships to build a reliable support network?

Make sure you implement your toolbox:

>> How will you remind yourself to utilize your tools when you're facing challenging emotions or situations?

>> Can you identify any potential obstacles to using your toolbox, and how might you plan to overcome them?

>> What will be your first tool when you need support, and why?

REMEMBER

In your quest for long-term sobriety, consistently using and implementing your carefully chosen strategies is a cornerstone of success. Sobriety is more than a milestone; it's a continuous journey with big triumphs and lengthy trials. By turning to your personal toolbox — the mindfulness practices that ground you, the physical activities that strengthen you, the creative expressions that free you, and the supportive community that sustains you — you are resilient against the many temptations of picking up and drinking. Remember that each tool you've gathered serves a purpose and is there for you when challenges arise. As you walk this path, know that your daily commitment to these strategies and your adaptability and willingness to seek help when needed will pave the way to a fulfilling and sober life.

What does emotional regulation look like for you?

The endeavor to regulate emotions is huge; it's an essential ingredient of achieving and maintaining long-term sobriety, and its effectiveness is supported by scientific research. Emotional regulation isn't about stifling your feelings; it's about managing emotions in a way that contributes to your well-being. Studies show that improved emotional regulation is linked to better mental health outcomes and can decrease the likelihood of relapse in individuals with substance use disorders (SUDs).

For example, a 20-minute mindfulness practice is more than a buzzword; it's a scientifically backed approach that activates the brain's prefrontal cortex, the region associated with higher-order brain functions such as awareness, concentration, and decision-making. By cultivating mindfulness, you are essentially rewiring your brain to handle stress more efficiently, as evidenced by neuroimaging studies demonstrating altered brain activity and improved emotional regulation in those who engage in regular mindfulness exercises.

Besides mindfulness, cognitive-behavioral strategies offer another scientifically validated pathway for emotional regulation, vital for navigating the complex terrain of sobriety. Cognitive-behavioral therapy (CBT) techniques equip individuals with the skills to identify and alter negative thought patterns that contribute to emotional distress. By challenging and reframing irrational or maladaptive thoughts, you can transform the emotional landscape of your experiences. This reconfiguration is not only about changing your thoughts but also about changing the emotional responses that stem from them.

The practice of cognitive restructuring is a key component of CBT that can be used to address the cognitive distortions that often lead to intense emotional reactions that may lead to picking up a drink. This technique teaches you to dispute and replace detrimental thoughts with more balanced, factual representations, which can lead to more regulated emotional responses.

Embrace science-backed approaches to emotional regulation as a part of your ongoing pursuit of sobriety. Explore various techniques to discover what works best for you, and commit to incorporating them into your routine. Emotional regulation might just look like a blend of acknowledgment, understanding, and action that ensures you live not at the mercy of your emotions but in harmony with them.

How to create effective communication in times of emotional turmoil

Communication can become particularly prickly when your emotions are running high. You may think you're expressing yourself clearly, but often, your message is muddled by the intensity of your feelings. By writing down your thoughts first, you can get a clearer idea of what you really want to say. This practice can help to distill true concerns and desires, preventing us from getting caught up in the heat of the moment.

When dealing with others, creating a "pause" before responding can transform interactions and relations. This pause is a space where you can check in with yourself, breathe, and consider how best to communicate your thoughts. Remember that effective communication is a two-way street; it's as much about listening as speaking. Show compassion — not only to others but to yourself as well. Allow your vulnerability to show because, in that space, authentic connections are made, and true healing can begin.

Building Emotional Resilience

As you continue to embark on the road to sobriety, you will inevitably encounter newfound emotional terrain. In this vivid and intense realm, shadows of previous struggles are brought to light amidst the myriad challenges of the present. This transformation is not solely about cultivating traditional concepts of strength or navigating the dichotomy of right versus wrong. It is about developing an adaptive and supple emotional stance to ride the crests and troughs of the sober life.

Research supports the idea that optimal stress response is a hallmark of resilience. Individuals who demonstrate a robust stress response tend to exhibit resiliency, while those with a blunted response may be at higher risk for relapse and continued substance abuse. This suggests that building resilience involves nurturing a healthy, responsive stress reaction.

Additionally, psychosocial rehabilitation, such as group therapy or programs like Alcoholics Anonymous, plays a critical role in constructing this resilience. Although relapse rates can be significant, failures are often seen as learning opportunities and steps toward complete abstinence.

According to a conceptual model that examines the impact of stressful childhood events on emotional and behavioral responses, it is understood that life experiences are processed through frontal limbic structures — including portions of the limbic system and the prefrontal cortex — which are highly adaptable based on the person's experiences. This underscores the importance of interventions that can reshape coping behaviors and enhance resilience.

REMEMBER

In the context of long-term sobriety, these insights affirm the necessity of embracing a dynamic form of emotional resilience.

Recognize and embrace your vulnerability as strength

In early recovery, it may feel as though the floodgates of suppressed emotions suddenly burst open, leaving you to navigate feelings that you've spent years numbing with substances. Embracing vulnerability does not mean being weak; acknowledging your emotions is fundamental to human experience. The bravery to admit and feel your weaknesses lays the groundwork for authentic growth and healing. It's about understanding that feeling emotions profoundly is not an intrinsic flaw but a testament to your humanity and a source of strength.

Learning to vocalize these emotions and be transparent about them with others is key. This openness fosters powerful relationships and community support, providing a scaffold to lean on as you face life's adversities. Rather than retreating into isolation, which may feel safe, engaging with others brings your internal struggles into perspective and bridges the gap between solitude and healing connections.

REMEMBER

Important! Dedicate a quiet moment each day for journaling. Make it a routine, perhaps in the morning, to set the tone for the day or in the evening to reflect on the day's events.

TIP

Reflective journaling will encourage you to engage with your emotions deeper by reflecting on and writing about your experiences, thoughts, and feelings. Here's how to incorporate reflective journaling into your recovery process:

>> **Choose a comfortable space:** Find a place where you feel at ease and free from interruptions. This could be a cozy corner in your home or a peaceful outdoor setting.

>> **Start with a prompt:** Begin each journaling session with a prompt that invites vulnerability. For example, "Today, I felt the most vulnerable when. . ." or "A situation that challenged my emotions today was. . ."

>> **Write freely:** Allow yourself to write without judgment. Express your emotions, fears, and challenges, as well as the moments of strength and joy. Don't worry about grammar or structure; focus on pouring out your thoughts.

>> **Reflect on your growth:** After writing, take a few minutes to read what you've written and reflect on the insights gained. Notice any patterns or recurring themes that emerge.

>> **Identify supportive actions:** Think about what actions you can take to address your vulnerabilities positively. This might include contacting a friend, attending a support group meeting, or practicing a specific coping skill.

>> **End with gratitude:** Conclude each journaling session by writing down one thing you're grateful for. Gratitude can shift your perspective and remind you of the positive aspects of your life.

>> **Review periodically:** Review your journal entries periodically to see how far you've come. Use it as a tool to recognize your growth and resilience over time.

REMEMBER

Making reflective journaling a regular part of your recovery journey creates a safe space to explore and understand your vulnerabilities. This practice is not to be missed; it's critically important. This process strengthens emotional regulation and fosters a sense of self-compassion and self-awareness for sustained sobriety.

Defining the significance of self-compassion in recovery

Self-compassion emerges as a pivotal element in your arsenal of emotional resilience, particularly within the context of your long-term recovery from substance use disorders. It embodies an empathetic and forgiving approach to oneself, especially when facing setbacks or challenges. The recovery journey is replete with potential stumbles, and it is essential to recognize that these instances are natural and intrinsic to your process. Recovery should not be misconstrued as a straight trajectory toward an end goal but as a multifaceted expedition rich with teachable moments.

The evidence supporting the role of self-compassion in recovery is compelling. Researchers Neff and Germer have reported a positive correlation between self-compassion and psychological well-being, suggesting that a kind attitude toward yourself can facilitate coping with difficult emotions and experiences. Additionally, a study in the *Substance Abuse* journal indicates that individuals with higher levels of self-compassion are less likely to turn to substances as a coping mechanism, reinforcing the protective nature of self-compassion in recovery.

Engaging in self-compassion involves cultivating a supportive inner dialogue that encourages rather than criticizes and emphasizes growth over the pursuit of unattainable perfection. This inner voice of kindness is a steadfast defense against the severe self-criticism that frequently arises with setbacks and relapses.

Implementing self-compassion into your recovery toolkit means ensuring that you have practical strategies ready for when you may confront feelings of inadequacy or failure. Positive self-talk is often employed here — replacing negative or self-defeating thoughts with affirmations of one's worth and acknowledging the progress made. Examples of positive self-talk might include statements like "I am more than this moment of struggle" or "Every step, no matter how small, is valuable."

Research published in the *Journal of Rational-Emotive & Cognitive-Behavior Therapy* finds that engaging in self-compassion exercises can significantly reduce the emotional distress associated with difficult experiences. That capacity to navigate negative emotions without devolving into a downward spiral is a testament to the practical power of self-compassion.

REMEMBER By integrating self-compassion into the fiber of your recovery journey, you are better equipped to manage the bumps along the way and transform potential obstacles into stepping stones for personal development and long-term success in maintaining sobriety.

Identifying emotional sobriety and adaptability

Emotional sobriety takes time and is about achieving a state of emotional stability wherein you're not easily capsized by life's challenges or the behaviors of others. It's understanding that you can influence how you react to negative situations — the ability to pause, reflect, and choose a measured response. Being emotionally sober means you don't allow your peace to be easily disturbed; instead, you foster adaptability, able to adjust your emotional sail no matter the wind's direction.

Developing this kind of emotional intelligence requires practice. It includes identifying physical reactions to your emotions and creating a space between feeling and reaction. Simple yet profound techniques such as mindfulness, meditation, and breathing exercises can anchor you in the present and prevent rash decisions spurred by raw emotions. It's about being proactive rather than reactive, acknowledging the full spectrum of your feelings without letting them define your actions.

By fortifying your emotional resilience through vulnerability, self-compassion, and adaptability, you become better equipped to face all life ahead of you.

REMEMBER Facing your emotions head-on is pivotal at any stage of your sobriety; it's the path to reawakening and growth. Like Lawrence, identify and confront your personal downfalls with courage — it's not weakness; it's ownership of your story. You've got this!

Chapter 4

Developing Long-Term Sobriety

The journey to long-term sobriety is as unique as you are, sprinkled with its own set of challenges and noteworthy achievements. The strength of your recovery hinges on a cornerstone that may not always be at the forefront of your thoughts — a solid support network. It's the people who offer a shoulder to lean on, the professionals who guide your insight, and the peers who walk the path alongside you. Understanding that recovery isn't a solo venture is crucial, and your ability to cultivate a network of supportive and understanding people can be a game-changer. Your sobriety is a composition of compassion and resilience, with each individual and support group contributing to your life's overall strength and vibrancy.

In this chapter, you will master creating a robust and varied support system that is dependable and tailored to your needs. You will learn to identify and engage with those who encourage you and provide comfort during challenging times. The chapter will guide you through navigating the supportive community of Alcoholics Anonymous as well as fostering close, empathetic relationships with individual confidants. You will understand how to integrate these various forms of support into a comprehensive network that strengthens and enriches your personal path to recovery, ensuring a variety of insights and experiences that keep you on track for continuous long-term sobriety.

Building a Solid Support Network

Embarking on the path of long-term sobriety, establishing a solid support network is beneficial and necessary for enduring success. This foundational aspect of recovery encompasses creating connections with those who genuinely understand the challenges and triumphs of sobriety. It's about surrounding yourself with people who can offer insight, encouragement, and accountability when needed. As you construct this network, you actively engage with peers, mentors, and support groups that align with your journey's goals, fostering a community that sustains and uplifts you every step of the way. This chapter will illuminate the strategies to build and nurture these vital connections, ensuring you have the strength of a collective behind you as you forge ahead in your sober life.

Find a reliable support system

Finding a reliable support system is akin to constructing a safety net that catches you when you stumble. It's about connecting with organizations and individuals who can relate to your struggles and remain steadfast in your triumphs. Ask yourself, "Where can I find a community that understands what I'm going through?" Alcoholics Anonymous (AA) and similar recovery networks (alcohol-free groups) offer more than just meetings; they are a source of collective wisdom and enduring hope. Engaging with such groups provides you with the scaffolding needed to build your new, sober life.

Your support system should be as diverse as it is strong, including professionals and peers who can guide and learn from you equally. It thrives on a foundation of mutual respect and shared experiences. Besides formal groups, look to trusted friends, family, or even co-workers who encourage positive change. If your goal is to survive and thrive in recovery, your support system must be multifaceted and reliable.

Developing a reliable support system is like laying the groundwork for a sturdy structure to support your sobriety journey. It's about seeking connections with people and organizations that truly understand your challenges and are unwavering in supporting your successes.

TIP

To strengthen your understanding of who and what can comprise your reliable support system, consider the following exercise:

1. **Create a support network inventory:** List individuals and organizations that have the potential to support your recovery journey. Include personal contacts, such as family and friends, and professional resources, such as counselors, support groups, and recovery programs.

2. **Identify shared values:** Reflect on the values and principles that matter most to you in your pursuit of sobriety. Seek out individuals and groups who align with these values, as they are more likely to provide the authentic, unwavering support you need.

3. **Offer mutual support:** Develop a plan to offer support in return to some members of your network while also considering what support you'd like to receive. This exercise underscores the reciprocal nature of support and the importance of a balanced exchange in relationships.

4. **Establish a contact plan:** Deliberately outline how you will engage with various support network members. This may include scheduling regular check-ins, making plans for social activities, or attending support group meetings.

By actively engaging in these exercises, you can better understand the components of a reliable support system and tailor your support network to meet your unique needs and aspirations in recovery. This deliberate, mindful approach can significantly enhance the effectiveness of your support system as you work toward long-term sobriety.

Peer Support: Who are you accountable to?

Peer support emerges as a critical and influential element of accountability, particularly in striving for long-term sobriety. It's important to identify who you're accountable to and understand that you're creating a woven group of shared accountability rather than a top-down structure.

Scientific evidence points to the decisive role that mutual support networks play in successful recovery programs. As someone on the path to sobriety, the concept of accountability extends beyond self-imposed discipline; it encapsulates a communal pledge to uphold the journey toward a common goal — *maintaining sobriety*.

The symbiotic relationship between peers seeking sobriety magnifies the power of accountability. You are not merely carrying the weight of your own commitment; you also become a cornerstone in another's foundation of sobriety. This shared responsibility and mutual support can significantly amplify your resilience and determination.

The principles of honesty and candor underpin accountability. The presence of individuals who approach you with compassionate directness, devoid of judgment, and whom you can reciprocate in kind is indispensable. This reciprocal commitment helps maintain focus and navigate the challenges accompanying the quest for long-term sobriety.

Genuine peer support does not recoil from challenging dialogues. Instead, it embraces them as essential components of the journey. These interactions encourage the confrontation and resolution of issues that might otherwise undermine the sobriety process. Thus, a network of peer accountability can serve as a critical scaffold, bolstering the entirety of one's sobriety endeavor.

In pursuit of your sobriety, the reinforcement of such a network is invaluable. Research highlights that an individualized approach to sobriety often benefits from social reinforcements, suggesting that the communal aspect of recovery can be as important as the personal commitment. A strong, honest, and mutually supportive peer group makes the path to long-term sobriety more attainable and resilient to potential pitfalls.

Peer support is a unique and potent form of accountability. As someone seeking sobriety, decide who you're accountable to. This doesn't suggest a hierarchy but rather a network of mutual responsibility. Having someone who shares the same goal of sobriety can be incredibly empowering. You are not just responsible for your own journey but also play a part in someone else's.

Accountability comes with honesty and openness. You need people who aren't afraid to call you out, with love and without judgment, and to whom you can do the same. It's the reciprocal promise to stay on course. Genuine peer support doesn't shy away from difficult conversations; it embraces them as necessary steps toward lasting sobriety.

TIP

Here's how to know if you're keeping company with the right people:

>> **You share your goals, and they remember:** You've laid out your plans, and the people in your corner listen and remember. They're who ask how your latest milestones are coming along and celebrate your wins, big and small.

>> **They're not afraid to have tough talks:** True pals aren't just there for the high-fives; they're ready to sit down and have those heart-to-hearts when the waters get choppy. They keep it real with you if they notice you're veering off course.

>> **You feel heard and supported, not judged:** When you speak, they're all ears — and heart. You don't get a wagging finger but rather an open hand. They understand the rough seas you're navigating and offer support rather than judgment.

>> **They encourage your progress, not perfection:** The people who truly have your back are the cheerleaders for your progress, not perfection-seekers. They're the first to remind you of how far you've come, not how far you must go.

>> **You want to reciprocate the support:** You know you're accountable to the right crowd when you're just as eager to return the support. The relationship is like a two-way street; you're each other's lookouts, ensuring everyone stays on the path.

REMEMBER

Having the right people by your side is like having a dependable safety system. They are your soft landing when life gets rough and the encouraging push that helps you regain your momentum. These individuals are more than mere spectators; they are active participants in your journey, deeply committed to the collective triumph over substance use disorder.

Nurturing healthy relationships

Long-term sobriety is sustained by nurturing healthy relationships. These are the relationships where we feel safe to be vulnerable without fear of judgment. It is the space where we can share our successes and our setbacks, knowing that both are met with understanding and support.

Develop nurturing relationships by being selective about who you surround yourself with — choose people who have your wellness at heart and those who lead by example. Spend time with those who uplift you and mirror the sobriety and personal growth you aspire to achieve.

Moreover, nurture these bonds by being present and engaged. Practicing mindfulness in your interactions can strengthen your connections with others. Listening actively, sharing joyfully, and participating genuinely contribute to your relationships' health. It's not merely about finding support but also about being supportive — thus creating a dynamic network where everyone flourishes.

Your support network is your stronghold on the road to recovery. It should bolster your willpower, mirror your determination, celebrate your victories, remain true to your course, embrace the community that embraces you, and watch as every step you take becomes a stride toward lifelong sobriety.

To engage in the principle of nurturing healthy relationships, I would propose an activity called "The Support Network Mosaic." This interactive exercise is designed to actively involve you in assessing and strengthening your current relationships, particularly those that contribute to your sobriety and overall wellness.

THE SUPPORT NETWORK MOSAIC ACTIVITY

Your objective is to create a visual representation of your support network that highlights the quality and strength of your current relationships while identifying areas for growth and development.

Materials required:

- A large piece of paper or poster board
- Markers, pens, or pencils
- Stickers or colored dots (optional)
- Magazines, scissors, and glue (for a collage approach, optional)

Instructions:

1. **Reflect and list:** Take a moment to reflect on the people in your life. List the names of individuals you consider part of your support network, including friends, family members, peers in recovery, mentors, or professionals.

2. **Categorize your relationship:** Next, categorize these individuals based on the type of support they provide. Use different colors or symbols to differentiate between emotional support, practical assistance, inspirational figures, accountability partners, and any other categories relevant to your journey.

3. **Create your mosaic:** Draw a large circle to represent yourself on your paper or poster board. Around this central point, arrange the names of your support network members near the center based on how nurturing and helpful the relationship is to your sobriety and growth. The closer to the center, the more significant their impact.

4. **Assess and analyze:** Reflect on the pattern that emerges. Are there clusters of supportive individuals? Are there areas that seem sparse? What does this mosaic tell you about the balance and health of your support network?

5. **Engage and expand:** Identify at least one relationship you would like to nurture further or a type of support you need

(continued)

(continued)

more. Make a plan to strengthen that connection or seek out new relationships that can fill any gaps.

6. **Share your insights:** If you're comfortable, share your mosaic with a trusted person in your support network. Discuss your findings and get feedback on how to cultivate these relationships further.

7. **Commit to action:** Finally, commit to one actionable step this week to nurture a healthy relationship in your life. It could be scheduling time with a friend, joining a support group, or expressing gratitude to a mentor.

By participating in this activity, you will have a tangible representation of your support network, gain insights into the health of your relationships, and set intentional goals to nurture connections crucial for your long-term sobriety. This exercise is more than just a reflective practice; it's about taking proactive steps to build a community around you rooted in mutual support and growth.

Mindful Lifestyle Choices

In this journey where maintaining sobriety is paramount, mindful lifestyle choices are the cornerstone for long-term success. It's not just about abstaining from alcohol or other substances; it's about crafting a way of life that nurtures you from the inside out and fortifies your resolve against the temptations and stresses that life throws your way.

What is mindfulness, and how do I get it?

Mindfulness is the art of being fully present and engaged in the moment, aware of our thoughts and feelings without getting caught up in them. How can one attain such a state? It begins with nurturing a deliberate focus on the present. This can be as simple as paying close attention to the food texture as you eat or the sensation of air entering and leaving your body as you breathe. It's about celebrating the mundane and finding depth in the simplicity of everyday life.

Cultivating mindfulness isn't an overnight feat. It's akin to building muscle — it takes consistent practice. Consider starting with meditation or deep breathing exercises. Dedicate a few minutes daily to sit in stillness, close your eyes, and simply notice your thoughts, letting them come and go. This practice can gradually extend into other areas of your life, helping you remain anchored in the present.

Integrating mindfulness into daily life

Embedding mindfulness into your daily routine can pull you out of the autopilot mode that we often default to. It's about making conscious decisions — choosing water over wine, a nutritious meal over fast food, or a walk instead of another TV show binge. Mindfulness can transform these choices from acts of denial to celebrations of self-care.

To integrate mindfulness, start by setting intentions for your day. Consider the kind of day you aspire to have and the personal interactions you wish to engage in. Mindfulness fosters a profound connection to your activities and the individuals around you. It allows you to see the bigger picture of your sobriety journey and recognize how each action shapes your path forward.

Routine can be a double-edged sword. On the one hand, it can provide a comforting structure and a predictable rhythm for your day. On the other, without mindful attention, your routine can become rote — flattening your life into a series of unexamined habits. Strike a balance by staying present even in repetitive tasks, and be willing to adjust established patterns that no longer serve your growth.

TIP

Skip to Chapter 15 to learn more about how to navigate your mindful practice and other mindful activities.

Balancing work and leisure in recovery

Recovery is an all-encompassing endeavor. It's a constant, delicate dance between work and leisure, where each step must be taken with intention. Remember that all work and no play can dull the spirit, but too much leisure can risk your hard-won discipline.

Work provides structure, purpose, and a means to contribute. Yet, it is essential to view work through the lens of recovery. It's not just about productivity — it's about engaging in meaningful tasks that resonate with your values and recovery goals. Choose work that invigorates rather than depletes functions that leave you with enough energy to enjoy your leisure time.

The activities you choose to fill your leisure time should refresh and delight you. This could include indulging in favorite hobbies, embracing physical activity, dedicating time to captivating projects, or immersing yourself in peaceful reflection. What's critical is that leisure during recovery reintroduces a sense of play into your existence. Through play, you'll find yourself infused with laughter, imaginative thinking, and bonding — all fundamental in crafting a rewarding and sober lifestyle.

Review the following collection of leisure activities tailored to your evolving needs in varying stages of your alcohol-free life.

REMEMBER

The key is to choose activities that resonate with personal interests and promote growth in all aspects of your life. It's essential to balance activities that provide relaxation and those that offer a sense of purpose and community connection. As challenges arise, these activities should serve as a foundation for maintaining sobriety and handling life with resilience and joy.

Balancing your sober life requires ongoing self-reflection and a willingness to pivot when the scales tip too far in one direction. Mindfulness plays a crucial role here, guiding you to notice when burnout looms or when idleness nudges you toward unwanted old habits. Listen to the cues of your body and mind — they are the wise messengers guiding your journey in sobriety.

Years 1-5 of sobriety

During the early years of your recovery, activities should focus on building stability, reducing stress, and fostering a sense of accomplishment.

>> **Mindfulness and meditation:** Helps manage stress and maintain a sense of inner peace.

>> **Yoga or Tai Chi:** For gentle physical exercise that promotes mental well-being.

>> **Art or music therapy:** Creative outlets that allow for emotional expression without substance use.

>> **Horticulture:** A way to nurture growth and enjoy a calming environment.

>> **Cooking classes:** Develop a new skill supporting Support a healthy lifestyle.

>> **Volunteering:** Give back to the community and create a sense of purpose.

>> **Group sports or activities:** For example, bowling or softball provide social interaction and physical activity.

>> **Learning a new language or instrument:** Positively challenges the brain.

Years 6-15 of aobriety

As you move into a more mature phase of sobriety, you can handle more complex or engaging activities that bring deeper fulfillment.

>> **Adventure sports:** Explore adventure sports like hiking, kayaking, or rock climbing for excitement and achievement.

>> **Advanced classes:** Take classes in personal or professional interest areas for ongoing intellectual development.

>> **Travel:** Exploring new cultures and environments can broaden your emotional, mental, and spiritual horizons.

>> **Mentorship:** Seek mentorship in personal growth.

>> **Community theater:** Engage in storytelling and connect with the local community.

>> **Home improvement projects:** Gain a great sense of accomplishment and build a comfortable living space.

>> **Spiritual retreats:** Explore faith or spirituality more deeply and seek unknown practices.

Over 16 years of sobriety

With significant time in sobriety, you might be ready for more challenging and self-reflective activities that prepare you for handling life's complexities.

>> **Pilgrimages or spiritual journeys:** Connect with a more profound sense of purpose and self.

>> **Writing a memoir or book:** Share personal stories of recovery and inspire others.

>> **Advanced educational pursuits:** What have you always dreamed of learning? Now is the time to obtain a degree or certificate in a field of passion.

>> **Philanthropy or community leadership:** Take on roles that shape and give back to society.

>> **Teaching or coaching:** Share your expertise with others, whether in recovery contexts or personal interests.

>> **Long-distance endurance activities:** It's time to go all in with your physical presence. Start training for marathons, cycling tours, etc., and this will test your physical and mental resilience.

>> **Political advocacy or activism:** Have you learned that you are passionate about making systemic changes related to addiction and recovery? Get involved, write letters, join a new party, and make a political stand.

>> **Art exhibitions or music performances:** Engage with the community and showcase your personal talents.

Drafting your sobriety blueprint

In the heart of a bustling city, Nora sat alone at her kitchen table, the room illuminated by the soft glow of early morning light. Today marked her sixth sober anniversary, an achievement that filled her with pride and melancholy. The journey had been arduous but fulfilling, yet now, she found herself on the precipice of an unexpected challenge — a divorce that threatened the stability she had so diligently built for herself and her two children.

As Nora sipped her coffee, she resolved not to let this personal storm compromise the foundation of her sobriety. She crafted a "sobriety blueprint," a proactive plan to fortify her against the tensions ahead. With a steady hand, she began to pour her thoughts onto paper, detailing her *triggers, potential stresses, and the concrete action steps* she would take to safeguard her hard-won sobriety.

Following is Nora's sobriety blueprint and action plan:

1. Identify triggers and stresses:

- Divorce proceedings that could evoke strong emotions and temptations to seek comfort in old habits
- Concern for her children's well-being, leading to overwhelming stress for them all
- Loneliness or feelings of failure as a partner

2. Outline coping strategies:

- Regular attendance at support group meetings to reinforce her commitment and gain invaluable perspective from others
- Scheduled check-ins with her sponsor to discuss feelings and receive guidance when triggers arise
- Daily mindfulness practices to manage stress and stay grounded in the present

3. Foster a support network:

- Open communication with family and friends who support her sobriety
- Playdates and activities with other sober parents to stay connected and give children a sense of normalcy

4. Create a routine for stability:

- A consistent daily schedule that includes time for self-care, exercise, and relaxation
- Healthy meals and activities they can look forward to each week

5. **Set short-term goals for motivation:**

- Establish weekly personal milestones to foster a sense of achievement, such as learning a new skill or completing a project

6. **Emergency contacts and professional support:**

- Have a list of emergency contacts, including a trusted therapist, for immediate support
- Consult with a legal professional to understand her rights and maintain a clear picture of the divorce process

7. **Prepare responses to high-risk situations:**

- Script and rehearse polite refusals for offers of alcohol at social or stressful events
- Develop a list of sober responses to intrusive questions or stressful encounters related to her divorce

As she penned the final points of her blueprint, Nora felt a surge of empowerment coursing through her. This was her life raft, the plan that would ensure her sobriety remained intact through the trials ahead of her. With her blueprint complete, she planned to meet with her trusted friend and mentor, Julia.

Since early in Nora's sobriety journey, Julia has been a pillar of support. Together at her local café, they discussed the document. With Julia's experience and insight, they refined Nora's strategies, ensuring no stone was left unturned. They discussed contingency plans for particularly difficult days and brainstormed additional sources of support. Julia's unwavering belief in Nora's strength and determination bolstered Nora's confidence.

By the time they finished their coffee, Nora's blueprint had transformed into a robust action plan. It was not merely a document but a testament to her resilience and a declaration of her commitment to preserving the life she had rebuilt. Nora felt ready to face the coming challenges, her blueprint a constant companion reminding her of the proactive steps she could take.

Nora clung to her blueprint as the days unfolded and the divorce proceedings began. It was more than a plan; it embodied her resolve to weather the storm without sacrificing the sobriety she held dear. And with each step she took, she not only preserved her sobriety but also strengthened the foundation of the new life she was building for herself and her children.

Maintenance Skills

Cultivating skills for sustained sobriety is crucial in the journey toward lasting recovery. These tools and practices will support you as you navigate your sober journey. While the path is personal and varies for each individual, certain core principles are universally beneficial for sustaining your commitment to sobriety. Consider this section as your guide to embedding these principles into your daily life to foster continuous personal growth and resilience against the temptations of relapse.

Embracing a sober life demands more than just the initial commitment; it requires embedding the essence of sobriety into the very fabric of your daily life. This integration is where the art of maintenance comes into play, transforming transient motivation into a persistent way of living. Building a robust routine that includes deliberate mindfulness, reflection, and proactive goal-setting does just that. Regular self-assessment and adjustments to these goals ensure that your life's direction always aligns with your deepest values and aspirations. It's not just about abstaining from substance use; it's about thriving in your personal and professional life, fortified by the discipline and clarity that sobriety brings.

REMEMBER

Sobriety is a journey, not a destination. Every experience can serve as a lesson, propelling you toward continuous self-improvement. By harnessing the power of education and self-awareness, you foster resilience against the siren call of old habits. As you forge ahead, keep an eye on the horizon, where learning and growth await. Embrace each day as an opportunity to reinforce your commitment to sobriety while nurturing the relationships and support networks that offer a safe harbor. With these strategies in hand, you are well-equipped to maintain your sobriety, come what may, as you evolve and withstand the ever-present lure of relapse.

Continuous self-reflection and growth

Embarking on the journey of sobriety isn't a sprint; it's a marathon that requires an unwavering commitment to continuous self-reflection and growth. To maintain long-term sobriety, developing the reflective skills that help you evaluate your progress, understand your setbacks, and, most importantly, celebrate your victories is vital. This dedication to self-reflection is a cornerstone in creating a sustainable, sober life filled with personal and spiritual growth that goes beyond the absence of alcohol or substances.

Here is a powerful exercise that will not only allow you to visualize your journey of sobriety but also to recognize and celebrate the strength and resilience you have demonstrated throughout it. By chronicling your milestones, challenges, and victories, you create a tangible representation of your progression, a roadmap of perseverance and adaptability.

TIP

Next to each milestone, challenge, or victory, write down the specific coping strategies you used to navigate that period or the lessons you learned from the experience. This could be a particular therapy technique, the support of a loved one, a personal mantra, or an insight that has since guided you.

CREATING YOUR RESILIENCE MAP

Follow these steps to create your Resilence map:

1. **Prepare your materials:** Choose a large sheet of paper, a poster board, and some markers or pens of different colors. You may also want stickers, printed photographs, or other visual elements to make your map more engaging.

2. **Draw your timeline:** Draw a long, horizontal line representing your sobriety timeline, which will be the foundation of your map.

3. **Mark your milestones:** Reflect on your journey and mark significant milestones along the timeline. These can include the

day you chose sobriety, your first whole week, month, or year of sobriety, and any other moments that stand out to you as significant achievements.

4. **Identify challenges and victories:** Between and around these milestones, identify challenges you've faced and victories — times when you overcame obstacles or made essential realizations. Place these along the timeline, wherever they best fit chronologically.

5. **Highlight patterns:** As you create your map, you may notice patterns in how you've dealt with challenges or how specific strategies have been particularly effective. Use colored pens or markers to highlight these patterns.

6. **Reflect and analyze:** With your completed map in front of you, take a step back and reflect on your journey. What does your map tell you about your evolution through recovery? Are there strategies that work best for you? How can this knowledge inform your path forward?

7. **Update regularly:** Your resilience map is a living document. As you continue your journey, you will encounter new challenges and achieve new victories. Keep updating your map to reflect these experiences. It will serve as a visual diary of your resilience and growth.

This activity is not just an exercise in reflection; it is a celebration of your journey and a strategic tool for your continued success. Your resilence map will remind you of where you've been and empower you with the knowledge of how you've succeeded, which is invaluable as you navigate the road ahead.

Creating a daily practice and personal progress

Developing a daily practice is more than a routine; it's a covenant you make with your future self. It starts with mindful lifestyle choices — nourishing your body, getting adequate sleep, and engaging in regular physical activity. These may seem trivial, but they set a strong foundation for recovery. They enable you to build resilience against the triggers and stresses that previously led to substance use.

TIP

One simple habit is embracing the profound power of gratitude; it is the easiest and most impactful way to enrich your daily practice and accelerate your personal progress. Gratitude is a catalyst for transformation, a tool that will reinforce your sobriety and reshape your outlook on life with every conscious application.

The science behind gratitude

Research has consistently shown that practicing gratitude leads to measurable mental and physical benefits. Gratitude could reduce the frequency and duration of episodes of depression, suggesting a powerful complementary practice for recovery. Gratitude leads to increased well-being and reduced stress — essential ingredients in recovery.

Gratitude has even been linked with improved sleep patterns, which is particularly important for individuals recovering from addiction whose sleep cycles may have been previously disrupted. Gratitude may even reduce inflammatory biomarkers in patients with heart failure, indicating its potential for physical health improvement.

Setting up your daily gratitude practice

1. **Select your gratitude space:** Establish a special place to engage with your practice undisturbed — a sanctuary for reflection and appreciation.

2. **Schedule gratitude time:** Integrate gratitude into your daily routine at a set time. This consistency is vital for it to become a natural part of your life, just like any other habit.

3. **Maintain a gratitude journal:** Commit to writing down at least three things you are grateful for daily. Elaborate on *why* these things matter to you to deepen the experience of gratitude; this is so important for the practice.

4. **Use gratitude visualization:** Couple your journaling with a visualization practice, allowing you to fully immerse yourself in the sensation of thankfulness for each aspect of your life you're grateful for.

5. **Share your gratitude:** Whenever you can, express your gratitude to others. This act of sharing magnifies the benefits by enhancing your connections with others and amplifying your positive emotions.

6. **Embrace challenges with gratitude:** Cultivate the habit of finding something to be grateful for, even in adversity. This approach will enable you to maintain strength and optimism, regardless of the circumstances.

You will nurture a more resilient, optimistic, and fulfilling life by firmly establishing gratitude as a central component of your daily practice. This isn't merely an optional add-on to your routine; it's an indispensable facet of your continuous growth and recovery. Make gratitude your steadfast ally, and witness the unfolding of an enriched quality of life that radiates from within.

REMEMBER

Creating a daily practice also means carving out time for reflection — through journaling, meditation, or simply sitting quietly, contemplating the day's events. Reflection not only helps in recognizing patterns but also empowers you to celebrate small wins along your path. It affirms that every day sober is an achievement and that personal progress isn't only measured by the significant milestones and the seemingly minor, yet significant, daily acts of self-preservation and self-love.

Setting and adjusting long-term goals

In sobriety, long-term goals offer a vision — a lighthouse guiding you through the tempestuous seas that sometimes never seem to change. These goals, whether related to personal relationships, career aspirations, or personal development, provide purpose and direction. However, the art of setting goals isn't just about aspiration; it's also about adaptability. As you grow and evolve on your sober journey, it becomes necessary to reassess and adjust these objectives. What matters most isn't the rigid adherence to a plan but the ability to remain fluid and responsive to life's inevitable changes.

Setting goals during recovery transcends mere aspiration; it inherently embraces adaptability — recognizing that your journey will catalyze changes in perspective and need. Personal evolution is not just a byproduct but a cornerstone of recovery, invoking the necessity for regular reevaluation of long-term ambitions.

The science of adaptability in goal-setting

Neuroscientific research has underscored the importance of adaptability, particularly in goal-directed behavior.

Studies have revealed that the brain's prefrontal cortex, responsible for executive functions such as planning and decision-making, is also crucial in adapting to new situations. This adaptability is evidence of neuroplasticity, the brain's ability to reorganize itself by forming new neural connections throughout life.

Further supporting this concept, the research emphasizes that being adaptable in goal-setting is linked to improved psychological well-being. This is particularly relevant in recovery, where psychological resilience is paramount.

A dynamic approach to goals is supported by the principles of self-determination theory (SDT), which posits that human motivation is not just driven by the attainment of goals but by the need for autonomy, competence, and relatedness. When your goals are too rigid, they may impede these innate psychological needs, suggesting that flexibility is essential for sustaining motivation over time, as various studies have indicated.

Embracing a dynamic strategy

Therefore, in your recovery, it is not the unwavering adherence to the original blueprint of your goals that is most pivotal but the ability to navigate and adapt to life's inherent unpredictability. A rigid attachment to an initial plan is counterproductive. It can impede your capability to engage effectively with emergent opportunities or obstacles, potentially stalling progress.

By incorporating this evidence-based adaptive approach to your goal-setting process, you are aligning with scientific understanding and leveraging the total capacity of your brain's adaptability to forge a resilient path through recovery. This approach ensures that your goals remain congruent with your evolving values and current life circumstances, enabling you to cultivate a recovery journey that is as rewarding as it is enduring.

REMEMBER

Take a moment to gather your thoughts, and as you do, consider the scientific insights that advocate for adaptability in goal setting. Reflect on the resilience of your own mind, its neuroplasticity, and its capacity for continual learning and adjustment.

The Power of Reflective Writing in Sobriety

It's essential to anchor yourself with tools that continue to nurture growth and self-awareness. One such practice, reflective writing, stands out as a beacon of introspection — a process that transcends mere record-keeping of your daily life. Think of it as a conversation with your innermost self, a dialogue that reveals the depths of your resilience and the contours of your aspirations. As you prepare to engage in this intimate form of self-expression, set aside the external world's clamor and turn your attention inward. With pen in hand and an open heart, you're not just chronicling a journey — you're scripting a future where clarity and intention lead the way to a life of sobriety, purpose, and fulfillment.

As you write, your intentions for maintaining sobriety and for the life you are creating become crystallized. You can cut through the noise and confusion of everyday life and focus on what truly matters to you. This act of writing becomes a compass, helping to guide your decisions and actions in alignment with your sober vision.

Moreover, visualizing your future through reflective writing is not just an idle daydream but a powerful manifestation technique. By vividly detailing the life you aspire to lead, you effectively set the stage for your reality to unfold. The clarity gained from reflective writing illuminates the path ahead, enabling you to navigate your journey with purpose and resolve.

In essence, reflective writing is a sanctuary where you can explore your inner world, untangle complex emotions, and emerge with a renewed sense of direction. It is a cornerstone practice in the architecture of your recovery — one that supports the continuous construction of a meaningful and sober life.

TIP

Setting long-term goals is vital to sustaining a sober lifestyle. Here are a couple of exercises that you may find beneficial for setting such goals:

Reflective writing exercise

Take a minute now and sit in a quiet place and write out the answers to these questions:

1. **What are my values, and how does living alcohol-free align with them?** Here, the goal is to weave together the fabric of your core beliefs with the decision to abstain from alcohol. It's about seeing the big picture of who you are and how being alcohol-free is not just a choice but a reflection of your essence.

2. **How has my relationship with myself improved since eliminating alcohol from my life?** This question nudges you to explore the internal shifts that have taken place. It's like looking into the mirror and seeing not just a reflection but a glow that wasn't there before — a glow that comes from health, self-respect, and a renewed sense of self.

3. **What activities bring me joy, and how can I incorporate more into my life now that I am sober?** Beyond the absence of alcohol, a whole world of hobbies, passions, and little moments spark joy. It's about rediscovering and fanning those sparks into flames of happiness and fulfillment.

4. **In what ways has my body benefited from my alcohol-free lifestyle, and how can I continue to support its health and well-being?** Sobriety isn't just a mental or emotional detox; it's a physical one, too. Reflect on the transformation your body is going through and celebrate every milestone. And then think about how you can keep giving back to your body for all the hard work it's doing.

5. **What barriers have I overcome in my journey toward sobriety, and what have I learned from them?** Every mountain climbed is both a triumph and a teacher. This question allows you to honor your struggles, learn from them, and remember that you're stronger than you might have thought.

REMEMBER

In sobriety, setting and adjusting long-term goals serves as a steady beacon guiding you through the challenges of recovery. These objectives provide a sense of purpose and direction, whether about personal growth, career aspirations, or relationships. However, setting goals isn't static; it involves adaptability and flexibility as one progresses on one's sober journey. The ability to reassess and adjust long-term goals in response to life's inevitable changes is crucial for sustainable sobriety. While setting and adjusting these goals is important, remaining responsive to life's flux is equally essential. Reflective writing can be a beneficial exercise to clarify intentions, align values with the decision to live alcohol-free, explore personal growth, and celebrate the triumphs and the lessons learned along the way. This exercise not only aids in creating a vision for the future but also encourages a deeper understanding and appreciation for the journey toward an alcohol-free tomorrow.

2

Decoding the Elements of Addiction: Genetics, Environment, and Spiritual Dynamics

Chapter 5

Genetic Factors and Environmental Influences

L iving a sober life is an intentional and transformative process, one that allows you to rediscover and recover aspects of your identity that may have been diminished by alcohol use. Research has shown that genetics play a significant role in addiction, with about 50 percent of the risk for alcoholism attributed to genetic factors. This knowledge is not a sentence but a tool for empowerment, providing crucial insights to guide you in maintaining a life free from alcohol.

In this chapter, you'll dive into the relationship between genetics and substance use disorders (SUDs). The scientific evidence is revealing while genetics contribute substantially to the risk of addiction, they are part of a broader picture that includes environmental factors and personal choices. This understanding serves not as a limitation but as a foundation for developing personalized strategies that support your sober lifestyle, enabling you to live fully without the constraints of addiction.

Understanding Genetic Predispositions

The genetic underpinnings of addiction present a multifaceted picture, with research suggesting that genetics account for approximately 50 percent of the likelihood of developing alcoholism and between 30 percent to 80 percent for other substance use disorders. This chapter examines the critical influence of our genetic inheritance on the propensity for substance use disorders, identifies key genes implicated in these conditions, and explores how genetic testing can inform individualized approaches to recovery.

Exploring family history and genetic influences

Your family history provides a vital clue to your genetic predisposition to SUDs. Studies highlight a notable risk increase for individuals with first-degree relatives who have a history of SUDs. Nonetheless, separating genetic factors from environmental ones can still be challenging. Acknowledging your inherited risk can empower you to take preventative steps toward long-term sobriety.

When examining the roots of SUDs, your family history is a pivotal factor, providing valuable insights into your genetic predisposition. The evidence is compelling: children of substance abusers are twice as likely to develop substance abuse problems and three times more likely to develop addictions to substances such as ethanol or marijuana compared to those with unaffected parents. Such statistics underscore the hereditary nature of these disorders.

The familial aggregation of alcoholism, in particular, has been well documented; individuals with an alcoholic parent are five times more likely to develop alcoholism themselves. This strong familial link extends beyond alcohol to other drugs of abuse, where first-degree relatives of substance abusers also show higher rates of addiction. This suggests that the biological legacy of addiction is not substance-specific but rather a general predisposition toward addictive behaviors.

Despite the robust data underscoring the role of genetics, one of the main challenges in family-based studies is the intricate task of disentangling the genetic contribution from environmental influence. For instance, parental divorce or psychiatric disorders have been noted as environmental risk factors affecting the development of substance abuse in offspring. Such environmental variables can confound the precise interpretation of your genetic risk.

Further complicating the matter, research has indicated that while one's environment might influence the initial stages of drug use, the progression to full-fledged addiction is more deeply rooted in genetics. With genetic factors accounting for approximately 50 percent of the risk for alcoholism and varying from 30 percent to 80 percent for other drugs of abuse, the severity of SUDs seems to be particularly gene-dependent.

Despite the complexities, the growing understanding of genetic predispositions allows for more effective interventions. Acknowledging your inherited risk is not a sentence to a predetermined outcome but catalyzes empowerment. With this knowledge, you can take targeted, preventative steps toward sobriety. You can engage in early education, maintain vigilant awareness of substance effects, and develop coping strategies to mitigate risk. Exploring your family history and genetic influences is a scholarly pursuit and a practical tool in the lifelong journey toward health and sobriety.

Here are some suggestions for understanding your genetic predispositions:

TIP

>> **Map your family tree:** Create a detailed family health history, paying close attention to any instances of substance abuse or related disorders. Include as many generations as possible for a comprehensive view.

>> **Get your genetic blueprint:** Get a copy of your genetic blueprint through any of the recommended resources at the back of the book

>> **Seek genetic counseling:** Consider consulting with a genetic counselor who can guide you through understanding your family history and its implications for your health.

>> **Educate yourself:** Learn about the significant genes linked to SUDs and how they may affect brain chemistry and behavior.

>> **Be proactive with prevention:** Preemptively engaging in healthy lifestyle choices and stress-management techniques can be crucial if you have a known genetic predisposition.

>> **Stay informed:** Keep up to date with the latest research in genetics and addiction, as new discoveries may offer insights into personalized prevention and treatment strategies.

Following are some questions to ask yourself:

>> What does my family history tell me about my potential risk for SUDs?

>> What lifestyle changes can I implement to reduce the likelihood of substance abuse, given my genetic background?

>> How can I educate my family and loved ones about our shared genetic risks for SUDs?

>> How can I stay informed about new research on genetics and addiction?

>> How can I ensure that my approach to sobriety is personalized to my genetic and environmental context?

By asking these questions and implementing the tips provided, you will be better equipped to understand your genetic predispositions and take control of your journey toward long-term sobriety with a personalized and informed approach. Remember, knowledge is power, and in the context of recovery, it can be the key to unlocking a healthier and more fulfilling future.

Your genes matter — genetic links to substance use disorders

The genetic landscape of addiction is intricate, with specific genes being linked to the severity of substance abuse. Contrary to the initial stages of drug use, which are more influenced by environmental factors, the progression to addiction appears to have vital genetic underpinnings. This section will discuss the various genetic markers and their association with different substances, providing insight into how your genes can impact your sobriety.

Within the delicate interplay of your genes, specific genes have emerged as precursors of strength and vulnerability, influencing the severity of substance abuse. While your environment guides the early steps toward or away from substances, it is often your genetics that direct the journey toward addiction.

Scientists have discovered a risk locus on chromosome 5 linked to nicotine dependence, meaning you might be genetically predisposed to certain diseases and conditions.

Research often identifies these loci through association studies, where the frequency of certain genetic variants in individuals with a particular condition is compared with those without the condition. Identifying risk loci is important because it can help scientists and medical professionals understand the genetic factors contributing to diseases, leading to better diagnostics, treatments, and even preventative strategies tailored to individual genetic profiles.

It is also worth noting that genetic research continuously evolves, and findings related to risk loci are often specific to certain populations because genetic variations can differ across ancestries. Therefore, a risk locus identified on chromosome 5 may be part of complex interactions within the genome and influenced by environmental factors, making the study of these loci a critical aspect of research for those suffering from addiction.

TIP

Understanding your genetic predispositions can be empowering, but it's only one piece of the puzzle. To complement this knowledge, engage in holistic health practices that support your overall well-being, including a balanced diet, regular exercise, adequate sleep, and stress management techniques. Holistic health practices can help mitigate the impact of risk genes and enhance the genes that contribute to resilience.

Consider the genetic factors connected to substance use disorders as markers that point to the possibility of developing addiction. These genetic indicators are related to how your body processes substances and the functioning of your brain's reward system; in long-term sobriety, your brain's reward system will still need to be cared for and nourished.

Let's break this down into simple terms. RNA, or ribonucleic acid, is like a messenger in your body. It helps carry out the instructions that your DNA (your body's blueprint) gives to make proteins, which are the building blocks of everything in your body.

Now, there are special kinds of RNA called noncoding RNAs (ncRNAs) that don't make proteins but still have important jobs. They help control which genes are turned on or off, much like a light switch. Two important types of ncRNAs are microRNAs (miRNAs) and long noncoding RNAs (lncRNAs).

Here's why this matters for someone with addiction: MicroRNAs (miRNAs) are tiny managers. They make sure certain messages from your DNA don't get turned into proteins by either blocking them or breaking them down. Long noncoding RNAs (lncRNAs) are like the master controllers. They can change the structure of your DNA and control how it's read and used.

Research shows that these ncRNAs play a big role in how your brain reacts to addictive substances. For instance, when you use drugs, it can change the levels of these ncRNAs in your brain. This can affect how your brain's reward system works, which is the part that makes you feel pleasure and can lead to addiction.

Understanding these RNA molecules helps scientists figure out new ways to treat addiction. By knowing how these tiny managers and master controllers work, you can develop better strategies to secure your recovery for the long haul.

Understanding addiction mechanisms

By undertanding how certain molecules in your genetic structure affect addiction, you gain insight into the complex biological underpinnings of your addictive behaviors. This knowledge emphasizes that addiction is not a simple matter of willpower but is often a chronic condition driven by genetic and molecular factors.

» **Personalized approaches to recovery:** As addiction science evolves, RNA-sequencing technologies could lead to more personalized strategies for recovery. Understanding individual patterns of ncRNA expression might help tailor treatment plans more effectively for specific genetic profiles.

» **Potential for new therapeutic targets:** By understanding the role of ncRNAs in addiction, researchers are likely to identify new targets for therapeutic intervention. In the future, you might see treatments that modulate the expression or function of specific ncRNAs to help maintain long-term recovery.

» **Hope for progress:** Knowing that ncRNAs are currently being studied and that there is an expected improvement in understanding addiction-related abnormalities brings hope. Progress can lead to breakthroughs that will benefit all those in recovery!

» **Empowerment through education:** Educating yourself about the biological aspects of addiction, including the role of ncRNAs, empowers you to take an active role in your recovery process. Understanding the science can help you make informed decisions about your health and maintain a recovery-oriented mindset.

You can develop preventative treatment plans tailored to your needs by leveraging your genetic insights. Gaining insight into your genetic predispositions toward addiction is not only about identifying potential weaknesses; it's also about recognizing your capacity for resilience and recovery. It enables you to craft a path to recovery informed by your past experiences, current situation, and future goals. Your genetic information guides you on the path toward overcoming addiction.

EXAMINING A PERIOD OF RISK THAT EMERGES: 15 YEARS INTO SOBRIETY WITH DAVID

Over the past 15 years, David built a life of sobriety that has profoundly transformed him. Through tireless dedication, he has managed to turn his experiences with addiction into lessons that have fortified his resolve. He has built meaningful relationships, found fulfillment in helping others, and carved out a place where his voice and story inspire those grappling with similar challenges. His sobriety has been a steady foundation upon which he's constructed a stable and respectable life with two kids and a wife.

David's journey encountered an unexpected turn when he casually dipped his toes into the world of gambling. What began as harmless entertainment with small bets on sports events and the occasional lottery ticket slowly morphed into something more concerning. The initial excitement of a win started to fuel a familiar sensation — the rush, a potent reminder of his past addictive behaviors. As time passed, the frequency of these bets increased, and the amounts wagered grew larger. The adrenaline rush with each bet began to fill a void he hadn't known existed, and his cycle of risk and reward escalated.

He found himself confronted by an insatiable pull for gambling; David felt the firm ground he'd stood on for so many years begins to tremble. As the stakes of his bets rose, so did his awareness of the dangerous path he was treading — a path he had consciously avoided since embracing his sober life.

The situation forced David to confront the reality that the challenges of addiction are multifaceted and that the struggle for control does not end with abstinence from substances alone. It illuminated the importance of continued vigilance in *all* aspects of his life and the necessity to recognize and guard against *any* behavior that could trigger the cyclical nature of addiction.

Through this realization, David grasped that his sobriety entailed more than just staying away from alcohol and drugs — it meant actively maintaining a lifestyle that prioritized his mental and *emotional* well-being, avoiding pitfalls that could potentially unravel the fabric of his recovery. The discipline and self-awareness he had carefully used over the past 15 years were tested.

Mike's trainer introduced him to the simple idea of how vital his DNA may be in looking for optimal health. He became fascinated with his health. A huge night arrives with a bet; considering going all in on a high-stakes game, a part of him knows he's courting disaster. The compelling urge feels eerily similar to his old cravings for a drink. David begins to sense that the same genetic underpinnings that made him vulnerable to substance abuse might also be at play in this new compulsion.

David pauses and engages in deep introspection. He realizes that he's been here before in a different guise. The behavior might differ, but the pattern is the same — a repetitive, compulsive search for an external stimulus to provide a fleeting sense of reward.

As he contemplates his next move, David revisits his knowledge of lncRNAs and miRNAs. He understands that these molecular players could be impacting his neural pathways, potentially influencing his behavior toward seeking reward. He recalls Mike's research suggesting that changes in gene expression, possibly mediated by ncRNAs, can alter an individual's response to risky behaviors, just as they do with addictive substances.

The clarity profoundly alters his actions. David realizes that he is vulnerable not just to substances but to any behavior that can hijack his brain's reward system. This genetic insight empowers him to take the following steps:

1. **Reflect and acknowledge** He recognizes the familiar patterns of addiction, acknowledging that gambling is becoming more than a pastime — it's a risk to the foundation of his sobriety.

2. **Seek knowledge:** He educates himself further about the genetic risks for addictive behavior, solidifying his understanding of his vulnerabilities.

3. **Reaffirm his commitment to recovery:** David decides to recommit to sobriety, understanding that it extends beyond abstaining from substances — it's about maintaining control over all compulsive behaviors.

(continued)

(continued)

4. **Schedule professional consultation:** Knowing the significance of early intervention, he schedules a meeting with a counselor who specializes in addictive behaviors to devise a prevention strategy.

5. **Make lifestyle adjustments:** David begins to establish safeguards, such as financial limits and self-exclusion from gambling sites, and he commits to engaging in healthier activities that provide a sense of fulfillment and reward.

Through a *moment of clarity* and a dedication to understanding the genetic aspects of addiction, David navigates away from the problematic path of gambling. His story is of ongoing vigilance, underpinned by the sophisticated knowledge of genetic influences on behavior. It serves as a compelling reminder that the recovery journey is continuous and that scientific knowledge can provide tools to maintain resilience in long-term sobriety.

Your Genetic Roadmap to Recovery

The following exercise will help you understand your genetics and personalize your recovery strategies; you will identify potential risk factors and learn how to manage your recovery journey better.

1. **Educational foundation:** Spend 30 minutes researching the most commonly associated genes with alcoholism and substance use disorders. Focus on genes involved in alcohol metabolism, neurotransmitter systems, and reward pathways.

2. **Genetic marker identification:** Based on your research, list the genetic markers that are linked to alcoholism. Next to each marker, note whether it is related to metabolism, neurotransmitter systems, or other functions.

3. **Personal assessment:** With your list of genetic markers, consider if you have any symptoms or experiences that could suggest a genetic influence (e.g., unusually high tolerance, withdrawal symptoms, cravings).

4. **Discussion with health professionals:** Schedule an appointment with a genetic counselor or specialist to discuss your findings and get professional insights.

5. **Preventive actions:** Identify preventive strategies that could help mitigate the risks associated with your genetic predisposition. This could include lifestyle changes, therapies, or avoiding environmental triggers.

6. **Empowerment through education:** Commit to educating yourself *continually* about the genetic aspects of addiction. Subscribe to newsletters, follow research, or join support groups where genetics is a topic of discussion.

7. **Journaling:** Start a recovery journal where you track your thoughts, feelings, and behaviors about your genetic predispositions. Over time, this can reveal patterns you can address in your recovery strategy.

REMEMBER

Knowledge is a crucial aspect of your recovery. By exploring and understanding the genetic links to substance use disorders, you gain valuable insights into your personal journey toward long-term sobriety, allowing you to navigate it with greater confidence and control.

The role of genetic testing in long-term recovery

Genetic testing yields the potential for precise addiction interventions. By identifying genetic predispositions, you can receive personalized treatment strategies. This tailored approach enhances prevention efforts and improves recovery programs' effectiveness, ultimately leading to sustained sobriety.

Genetic testing stands at the forefront of modern addiction medicine, offering unprecedented precision in the formulation of intervention strategies. Identifying specific genetic predispositions opens the door to a realm of personalized treatment plans tailored to an individual's unique biological makeup. This level of customization is not merely an improvement but a revolution in the way we approach the prevention and treatment of substance use disorders.

Individuals equipped with the knowledge of their genetic vulnerabilities can work collaboratively with healthcare providers to craft a recovery program that anticipates and addresses potential challenges. For example, if a person carries genetic variants associated with a heightened response to stress, their treatment plan might include stress management techniques as a cornerstone of their recovery efforts.

Personalized treatment strategies incorporating genetic information can optimize medication selection, reduce the risk of adverse drug reactions, and adjust therapeutic approaches to align with an individual's genetic profile. The pharmacogenomics of addiction treatment is an emerging field where specific alleles may predict an individual's response to medications like naltrexone or methadone, which are used in the treatment of opioid and alcohol dependence.

The presence of genetic markers associated with addiction can serve as a powerful motivator for individuals in recovery. Knowledge of your genetic predisposition can engender a proactive stance toward health, prompting individuals to adopt lifestyle changes and engage more fully in their treatment programs. In this way, genetic testing does more than inform; it empowers.

Ultimately, your aim is sustained continuous long-term sobriety, and genetic testing is a critical tool in achieving this goal. It is not a panacea, but it promises longer-lasting recovery outcomes when integrated into a comprehensive treatment strategy. Genetic testing is the key to unlocking a future where addiction interventions are not just effective but enduring.

Impact of Environmental Factors

Environmental influences account for a considerable portion of addiction risk, with drug initiation heavily dependent on external factors. This chapter examines how early childhood experiences, peer influence, and stressors contribute to substance use and the importance of developing healthy coping mechanisms.

Let's analyze how they shape the landscape of addiction and the significance of proactive measures in fostering resilience.

The realm of environmental influences on addiction is vast and decisive. It is irrefutable that these external factors play a substantial role in the initiation and continuation of substance use. From the formative power of one's early years to the persuasive sway of peers and the formidable force of stress, the environment weaves a complex web that can entrap individuals into patterns of substance abuse.

At the earliest stages of life, the impact of childhood experiences sets the stage for later behavior. The seminal research on adverse childhood experiences (ACEs) has illuminated a direct correlation between childhood trauma and the probability of future substance use disorders. Children who experience physical, emotional, or sexual abuse, neglect, or household dysfunction, such as parental substance abuse or mental illness, are at a markedly increased risk for developing addiction. This early vulnerability underscores the necessity for intervention strategies that prioritize the mental and emotional well-being of children, aiming to disrupt the potential trajectory toward substance abuse.

As individuals progress into adolescence and young adulthood, the influence of peers becomes paramount. The desire for acceptance and fear of exclusion can drive impressionable young people toward substance experimentation and, potentially, into the clutches of addiction. Peer groups that normalize or encourage drug use can significantly alter an individual's perception of risk and reward concerning substances, making resistance to experimentation all the more difficult. It is essential to bolster young people with the self-confidence and social skills to make autonomous decisions, irrespective of peer pressure.

Stress is another omnipresent environmental factor with a direct link to substance use. Individuals who encounter high-stress environments, whether due to socioeconomic factors, work pressures, or personal relationships, may turn to drugs or alcohol as a maladaptive coping mechanism. The consistent or acute experience of stress can erode an individual's capacity for self-control, leading to reliance on substances for temporary relief. This connection between stress and substance use highlights the critical need for effective stress management techniques as a preventative and recovery-focused measure.

Developing robust, healthy coping mechanisms is paramount to combating these environmental risk factors. Teaching individuals how to navigate stress, build robust support systems, and seek out positive environments can significantly reduce the sway of environmental influences on substance use. Engaging in substance abuse prevention programs, fostering community support, and providing access to mental health services are concrete steps that can strengthen individual resilience and diminish the likelihood of addiction.

While environmental factors undoubtedly contribute to the risk of addiction, they also offer a blueprint for prevention and intervention. By understanding and addressing these influences, we can forge a path toward reducing substance use disorders and enhancing the prospects for long-term recovery.

Investigating early childhood experiences

Adverse childhood experiences (ACEs) have a profound impact on the risk of developing SUDs. The vulnerabilities introduced by childhood traumas can set a trajectory toward substance use as a form of coping. Through understanding this link, preventive measures and supportive environments can be strategized to mitigate this risk.

The correlation between ACEs and the subsequent risk of substance use disorders (SUDs) is both undeniable and profound. Extensive research has illuminated the stark reality that childhood traumas — such as emotional, physical, or sexual abuse; neglect; and household dysfunction like witnessing domestic violence or growing up with family members who suffer from mental illness or substance abuse — create vulnerabilities that can steer an individual's life path toward the misuse of substances. These experiences disrupt the brain's normal development and can lead to changes in the stress response systems, making self-regulation and handling emotional distress more challenging.

It is these vulnerabilities, often stemming from a sense of insecurity and unresolved psychological pain, that can lead individuals to seek solace in drugs or alcohol — substances that provide a temporary escape from the haunting effects of their traumas. However, by recognizing the inextricable link between ACEs and the development of SUDs, we can be proactive in breaking this cycle.

Preventive measures are not only necessary but imperative. Early intervention strategies — such as providing at-risk children with consistent, caring relationships and safe environments — can significantly alter the potential progression toward substance use. Programs that foster resilience and teach coping skills and emotional regulation can empower children to handle life's challenges in healthier ways.

Moreover, creating supportive environments where traumas can be addressed therapeutically is crucial. Children who have experienced ACEs require compassionate, trauma-informed care that acknowledges their experiences and provides the support necessary to heal and thrive. Schools, healthcare providers, and community organizations must be equipped to recognize the signs of trauma and respond effectively.

Investing in the well-being of children is investing in the future. Mitigating the risk of ACEs leading to SUDs is not merely a clinical objective; it is a societal imperative that can yield dividends in the form of healthier adults and communities. By understanding the link between early childhood experiences and substance use, we can develop strategies that not only prevent addiction but also enhance overall well-being for generations to come. The evidence is clear, and the time for action is now — let us commit to nurturing the resilience and recovery of those affected by childhood adversities.

How my peers influence me

The social environment, particularly during formative years, plays a critical role in substance use behaviors. Peer pressure and the desire for social conformity can lead to experimentation and, potentially, addiction. This section explores how relationships and social circles influence decisions regarding substance use.

When delving into the pivotal role of the social environment and its impact on substance use behaviors, it's imperative to acknowledge the immense sway of peer dynamics, especially during the critical formative years of an individual's life. The drive for social acceptance coupled with the potent force of peer pressure can not only nudge but outright propel young individuals toward experimentation with drugs or alcohol. If unchecked, it's a pathway that can spiral into the abyss of addiction.

During the journey from adolescence to adulthood, the influence wielded by peers is undeniable and often overpowering. It is a time when the opinion of friends and acquaintances can overshadow one's own judgment, steering behaviors and decisions in a bid for social conformity. Craving for acceptance and fear of rejection are acute during this period, making the temptation to align with the behaviors of one's social group intensely compelling.

Peer pressure can take many forms: the overt offering of a substance, the subtle glorification of drug use through conversation and behavior, or the silent weight of expectation to partake in what the group deems as normative conduct. For those who are on the precipice of adolescence, where identity is still malleable, these moments can define their relationship with substances for years to come.

This section doesn't just recognize the challenge; it sheds light on the mechanisms at play. Understanding how relationships and social circles can influence decisions about substance use is foundational to developing effective prevention strategies. When we grasp the power of social influence, we can begin to empower individuals with the skills needed to make autonomous choices, stand firm in their convictions, and seek peer groups that foster healthy behaviors.

Education programs focusing on self-esteem building, critical thinking, and assertiveness training can provide young people with the tools to resist peer pressure. Encouraging open dialogues about the realities of substance use and providing platforms for positive peer interactions can reinforce an individual's ability to make informed, independent decisions.

The goal here is clear: equip our youth with the resilience to navigate their social landscapes without succumbing to harmful pressures. When they realize that their worth is not contingent on group conformity, especially concerning substance use, we create a bulwark against the tide of addiction. It is paramount that young people feel supported to forge their paths, ones that lead toward their well-being and away from the risk of addiction. This understanding is not only crucial — it's transformative. When we stand firm against the undertow of peer influence, true autonomy, and healthier lifestyle choices emerge.

Stressors and coping mechanisms

Stress is a pivotal environmental factor in substance use and abuse. Individuals with deficient stress responses or maladaptive coping strategies may be more susceptible to addiction. This segment delves into the types of stressors commonly associated with substance use and emphasizes the development of effective coping strategies as a key component of prevention and recovery.

The relationship between how individuals respond to stress and the likelihood of turning to drugs or alcohol is well-documented and deeply concerning. Those who find themselves with inadequate stress response mechanisms or who resort to maladaptive coping strategies are, without a doubt, at greater risk of succumbing to the lure of addiction.

The spectrum of stressors that can precipitate substance use is broad and multifaceted, encompassing everything from the daily pressures of life and work to the profound impact of significant life changes or traumatic events. The link between these stressors and substance use is not simply correlative; it is causative. When individuals face overwhelming stress without the proper tools for management, they may seek immediate relief in the form of drugs or alcohol — a perilous path that can quickly lead to dependency and addiction.

REMEMBER

It is crucial to understand the types of stressors that are commonly entwined with the risk of substance use. Chronic stressors, such as ongoing financial hardship, job instability, and persistent relationship conflicts, create a relentless sense of unease that can erode an individual's resolve over time. Acute stressors, including the sudden loss of a loved one, natural disasters, or a personal health crisis, can precipitate a rapid descent into substance use as individuals grapple with intense emotions and the disruption of their lives.

In the face of these stressors, developing effective coping strategies is a foundational element of prevention and recovery. It is not an overstatement to say that equipping individuals with the tools to handle stress healthily is urgent. Teaching stress management techniques, such as mindfulness, relaxation exercises, and problem-solving skills, can fortify individuals against the temptation to turn to substances as a coping mechanism.

Emotional regulation, too, is a vital coping strategy. By learning to identify, understand, and manage their emotions, individuals can navigate stressful situations with greater composure and resilience, reducing the impetus to seek escape through substance use. Additionally, fostering strong social support networks provides an indispensable resource for individuals to lean on during times of stress, further diminishing the appeal of drugs and alcohol as a means of coping.

In sum, stress is an undeniable driver of substance use and abuse, but it is not an invincible one. By shining a light on the types of stressors that commonly lead to substance use and by emphasizing the development and reinforcement of effective coping strategies, we can significantly mitigate the risk of addiction. This proactive approach is not merely beneficial — it is essential in weaving a safety net of resilience that can catch individuals before they fall into the clutches of substance dependency.

Navigating Genetics and My Environment

The interplay between genetics and environmental factors shapes the risk and resilience to substance use disorders. Taking into account the intricate web woven by the interaction between genetics and environmental factors, it becomes clear that understanding this relationship is pivotal to addressing substance use disorders (SUDs). The final chapter of our exploration is dedicated to guiding readers through the complexities of this interplay and highlighting the importance of a tailored approach to achieving and maintaining sobriety.

The complex dance between our genetic makeup and environmental experiences dictates not only our physical attributes but also plays a determining role in our behavior, health, and susceptibility to addiction. It is critical to grasp that while 99.9 percent of our genetic material is identical to that of any other person, it's the remaining 0.1 percent that engrains our individuality and influences how we navigate the world — how we metabolize nutrients, how our cardiovascular system functions, and even how we may be predisposed to certain diseases, including SUDs.

Behavioral genetics researchers clarify the distinction between gene-environment correlations, which describe how our genetic predispositions can shape the environments we encounter, and gene-environment interactions, which reflect how our genes can dictate the degree to which specific environmental influences affect us. These concepts underline the multifaceted nature of addiction, where both our inherited traits and life experiences shape our physiological and psychological responses to potential stressors or drugs.

In this dense jungle of genetic and environmental interplay, it is evident that a one-size-fits-all approach to prevention, intervention, and recovery from substance use disorders is inadequate. The nuanced understanding of gene-environment interactions equips us with a powerful lens through which we can view addiction — helping us to see beyond the surface and to appreciate the unique constellation of factors contributing to each individual's journey with substances.

Advancements in genomics, such as genome-wide association studies and the development of polygenic scores, are beginning to illuminate the path ahead. These tools may enable more precise predictions of how specific genes and environmental experiences can forecast an individual's well-being. This knowledge could transform our strategies for preventing and treating addiction, allowing us to tailor interventions unique to each person's DNA code.

Understanding your genetic blueprint and how it interacts with environmental factors is crucial. Through this personalized lens, one can navigate the path toward sobriety with greater clarity and confidence, acknowledging that the road to recovery is paved with bespoke stones, each carved by the hands of our genetic and environmental history.

Recognize the combined impact on substance use

Combining genetic predisposition with environmental risks paints a more complete picture of addiction complexities. Recognizing both elements allows for a more comprehensive approach to addressing substance use, considering all aspects of an individual's life and history.

When we consider the combined impact of genetics and environmental factors on substance use, we gain a more nuanced and complete understanding of the complexities inherent in addiction. This integrated perspective is essential for a comprehensive approach to addressing substance use, taking into full account all aspects of an individual's life and history.

Family-based studies have shown that children of substance abusers are significantly more likely to develop substance abuse and addiction compared to those with unaffected parents, highlighting the role of genetics For instance, adult first-degree relatives of individuals with an addiction to drugs such as opiates, cocaine, cannabis, and ethanol are at an eightfold increased risk of SUDs.

However, distinguishing the contribution of genetic variance from environmental factors remains challenging. Intriguing evidence from animal studies reveals a complex interplay between genetics and environment. For example, a study showed that male rats with a history of cocaine self-administration could sire offspring more susceptible to cocaine cues, suggesting that both hereditary and environmental factors play a role in the propensity for addiction.

The integration of studies on individual variations in genome sequences with these observations aims to understand how an individual's risk or resistance to an addiction syndrome is mediated. It is hoped that this will lead to the identification of biomarkers for susceptibility and resilience to addiction, providing novel therapeutic targets for improved treatment of addiction syndromes. Individuals with addiction have a strong desire to quit. Still, successful treatment and recovery rates are low, emphasizing the need for personalized approaches in the face of genetic and environmental influences.

Ultimately, recognizing the combined impact of genetics and environment on substance use leads us to appreciate that each person's path to addiction, and consequently their route to recovery, is distinct. This recognition underscores the necessity of personalized approaches in the prevention, treatment, and management of substance use disorders. By accounting for the intricacies of each individual's genetic makeup and environmental experiences, we can better tailor interventions, support mechanisms, and treatment plans that are most likely to result in successful outcomes for those striving to achieve and maintain sobriety.

Have a personalized approach to recovery

Personalized recovery is imperative. Individuals can work alongside healthcare professionals to create a tailored recovery plan by embracing one's genetic makeup and environmental history. Personalized recovery strategies cater to specific needs and increase the likelihood of long-term success and sobriety.

The journey to recovery is unquestionably an intimate and personal endeavor that must be tailored to fit each individual's unique genetic makeup and life experiences. To embark on a path to sobriety that is both successful and enduring, it's essential to have an approach to recovery that addresses the individual's specific needs, challenges, and strengths.

Your recovery journey must be as unique as you are. This message resonates with the understanding that no two individuals share the same genetic predispositions, environmental influences, or life stories. As such, recognizing the need for a personalized recovery approach is not just wise — it's imperative.

In discussions about personalized recovery, the concept of Bio-Individual Nutrition is often mentioned. This approach recognizes that there is no one-size-fits-all diet; instead, it's about understanding the science and thought process behind various therapeutic diets and customizing them to avoid pitfalls while enhancing your health and well-being. Using cutting-edge tools like symptom cluster lists and food sensitivity categories, you can streamline a recovery approach that considers your body's unique responses to different substances and lifestyle choices.

Physical activity also plays a significant role in recovery, as demonstrated by testimonies of individuals who have found their optimal rhythm in exercising certain days with interspersed rest days. This kind of fine-tuning is critical for maintaining physical health and mental resilience in recovery.

Furthermore, recovery is not solely about the physical aspect. It encompasses your spiritual and emotional well-being. Mindfulness and meditation practices can play an integral part in supporting these facets of your recovery, particularly if you possess genetic variations that affect stress responses or emotional regulation.

It is also important to recognize that the knowledge of your genetics can be transformative. Understanding your genetic predispositions can help you make more informed decisions about your recovery process. For example, if you have a genetic sensitivity to certain substances, this might influence your approach to managing cravings and triggers.

For many, recovery is not just about abstaining from substances but about discovering or rediscovering a sense of meaning and direction in life. A personalized approach to recovery involves exploring what brings you joy and fulfillment and finding ways to integrate these elements into your daily life.

Understanding and honoring your individuality when navigating the complexities of recovery is essential. By taking a personalized approach that considers your genetic predispositions, environmental factors, nutritional needs, physical activity preferences, and emotional and spiritual well-being, you can create a recovery path that is as effective as it is personal.

Recovery is not just about surviving. It's about thriving, unleashing your self-preservation, and living your ultimate life — one step at a time.

Chapter **6**

The Spiritual Dimension of Recovery

magine stepping into a world where essence feels lighter, grounded in a clear and far-reaching purpose. You're about to embark on a journey within, examining an area of your life that's as crucial as it is often overlooked — your spiritual health. Recognizing the signs of spiritual sickness is akin to feeling a void that even the finest earthly pleasures cannot fill. It's a disconnection from joy, a silent but deep sense of isolation that your achievements and possessions can't seem to bridge. It's the nagging feeling that you're utterly alone despite being surrounded by people — your sense of direction blurred and your inner peace disturbed.

In this chapter, you'll discover that tapping into your spirituality is not just an esoteric concept but a vibrant, essential part of total well-being that merits your attention and care. You'll learn to spot the subtle signs of spiritual malaise, understand its roots, and navigate the often-unseen impacts it can have on every facet of your life. This isn't about adhering to a particular creed or doctrine; it's about nurturing your spirit, aligning with your core values, and filling your life with purpose and authenticity. Uncover the transformative power of spiritual wellness and how it can light a path to a more connected, joyful, and alcohol-free existence.

Recognizing Spiritual Sickness

Over time, as you begin to peel away the layers of recovery, it becomes clear that sobriety is not just a physical state but a holistic one that includes your spiritual well-being. Recognizing spiritual sickness is a fundamental step toward achieving a balanced life. It involves tuning into a profound sense of disconnection, an emptiness that cannot be filled with substance, achievements, or possessions. You may notice that what once brought you joy now feels hollow or that relationships and endeavors that should be fulfilling leave you feeling more isolated than ever.

As you learn to identify the roots of your spiritual ailment, you'll discover that they often stem from everyday behaviors and experiences. These may include the absence of a daily spiritual practice, harboring unexpressed resentment, or the heavy burden of selfishness and egocentrism. Just as a body can suffer from the lack of proper nutrition, your spirit can wither without the nourishment of meaningful connections, the pursuit of core values, and dedicated time for reflection and self-discovery.

WARNING

The consequences of ignoring spiritual sickness can ripple through all facets of your life. Like an invisible weight, it can distort your interactions with others, leading to strained relationships and a pervasive feeling of dissatisfaction. On an internal level, your unaddressed spiritual malaise can manifest in a variety of unsettling ways — from chronic stress and anxiety to a total retreat from social situations, locking you in a cycle of negativity and despair. Recognizing and actively treating your spiritual sickness is therefore not just beneficial — it's necessary for authentic and lasting sobriety.

Recognizing spiritual sickness

You might find yourself enveloped in an inexplicable feeling of hollowness, as if a vital component of your being has been siphoned away, leaving you incomplete. This desolation can manifest as a profound sense of emptiness that grips your days or a pervasive lack of purpose that haunts your actions. You wander through life feeling disconnected, not just from those around you, but from yourself and your sense of direction. The joy in activities that once brought you happiness is dimmed, and you're left clawing for the light in the darkness of your own thoughts. This is what it means to be spiritually bankrupt; it's a deficit that cannot be reconciled by tangible means, but through nurturing your inner self.

Your understanding of spiritual health may need redefining if you find that negative emotions and a persistent sense of dissatisfaction continuously weigh you down. The internal compass that should guide you toward harmony and fulfillment inexplicably spins out of control, leaving you in a cycle of self-centeredness and distorted perception. Recognizing spiritual sickness comes down to an awakening — realizing that you're caught in a web of distorted thinking that skews your view of the world and yourself. The signs are in the patterns of isolation you impose upon yourself, the overwhelming selfishness that edges out empathy, and the nagging sense that you are irreversibly stuck in your current predicament.

To break free from spiritual sickness, it's crucial to undertake a journey of self-discovery and healing. The malaise of the spirit can often be a silent fight, but it is not one that you have to confront alone. Seeking guidance, whether it be through community, therapy, or spiritual practices, is the first step toward reclaiming your vitality and rediscovery of joy. Understanding that you might need the help of others to recognize the symptoms is part of the recovery process. As you begin to realign with your core values and strive toward a life filled with purpose and peacefulness, you'll notice the darkness recede, making way for a resurgence of that quintessential spark that defines your spirit.

THREEFOLD DISEASE WITH FELICIA

When I understood my alcoholism as a threefold disease, which means I have an obsession of the mind, a physical allergy, and a spiritual sickness. When I looked around at other people in the rooms who seemed to have lower bottoms than me (outwardly), I thought I didn't belong, and I questioned whether or not I was an alcoholic. Learning about spiritual sickness was what helped me realize my problem and has helped me to stay sober and seek spiritual wellness continually.

I know you might have squirmed when you read the word "alcoholic." If so, please don't stop reading because I'm so excited to explain why I'm grateful for being an alcoholic and how accepting this word kickstarted my healing from spiritual sickness. I had so much pride (and I probably still have remnants). And when I say pride, I'm not talking about the good kind. I'm talking about the "I'm-better-than-you, I-don't-need-your-help," kind of pride. The type of pride that made me think I was the center of the universe, the type of pride that edged God out of my life.

So, for me, taking on the identity of "alcoholic" was necessary to be humbled enough to break down the pride. It made me realize that I'm human, not better than anyone else and that I need you and my Higher Power. I have learned that being humbled by a power greater than myself is the anecdote of pride, which is also the anecdote to my ongoing spiritual sickness. As long as I continue to be human, there will be periods of spiritual sickness, so I must continue on my journey toward spiritual wellness.

What does spiritual wellness look like to me? It's about keeping myself right-sized and remembering that I'm not God. To do this, I spend time with my Higher Power by reading recovery literature and the Bible, praying, and meditating. Doing this introduces me more deeply to God and His character. I experience God's grace, love, and compassion through these encounters. I try to remember that I am created, not the creator. So, regarding my role, I have to ask my creator, "What did you create me for? Please use me the way you intended."

As long as I keep this posture, I am a little safer from being too proud and a little safer from relapse and spiritual sickness. — Felicia Hermle, an alcoholic living in long-term recovery

Defining spirituality

Spirituality infuses your being with a vitality that extends beyond the five senses, engendering a link with the universe that eclipses mere physical existence. This spiritual essence plants your feet firmly on the ground, enveloping you in a cocoon of serenity and purpose. At its core, your spirituality is the sanctuary where stillness meets the tumult of life, providing a tranquil center from which to navigate the stormy seas of the everyday.

Embracing spirituality empowers you with an inner fortitude, enabling you to engage with life altruistically and with clear intent. It is as if a quiet light within you illuminates your path, guiding you toward acts of kindness, peace, and generosity. This illuminated path leads you away from selfish behaviors, toward a broader horizon where community and shared experience become the anchors of your existence.

Research has consistently shown that spirituality and religious involvement are linked to better health outcomes. A review by Moody-Smithson (2001) prepared for the Center for Substance Abuse Treatment (CSAT) indicated that 90 percent of the studies they examined found substance abuse to be less common among more religious individuals. This aligns with the notion that spirituality imbues a sense of vital purpose and helps individuals resist the lure of substance abuse.

Further evidence points to the benefits of incorporating faith-based elements in treatment programs. For example, in a recently published study, it was observed that clients who completed 90-day treatment programs, including those with spiritual components, reported less substance use at follow-ups. This suggests that spirituality can offer an added layer of recovery support, strengthening one's inner fortitude to face challenges with clear intent and stay on a path free from substance dependence.

Investigations into the role of spirituality in moderating stress and substance use are particularly revealing. A recent study found that higher levels of spirituality correlated with lower substance use among high school students, even in the face of psychological stress. This provides tangible proof that the "tranquil center" offered by spirituality enables individuals to navigate life's "stormy seas" with greater calm and resilience.

Studies on various populations, including Indigenous youths and young black homosexual men, have emphasized that spiritual and religious engagement can both serve as a source of resilience and, conversely, may increase susceptibility to substance use due to associated stigma. This complexity underlines the idea that spirituality isn't a one-size-fits-all solution but rather a personal sanctuary where the effects can differ based on context and individual coping mechanisms.

Hundreds of evidence-based studies emphasize the positive impact of faith on health and well-being, a notion supported by extensive research from institutions like Duke University and various healthcare professionals. This extensive body of work validates the idea that by embracing spirituality, people can indeed become more altruistic, find peace, and contribute to their communities, moving away from egocentrism as their spiritual essence guides them.

Spirituality offers robust evidence that it can indeed infuse individuals with vitality, guide them with purpose, and enable them to engage with life in a more meaningful and generous way, as suggested by the initial definition.

REMEMBER

At the heart of the spiritual journey is your relationship with the intangible — those aspects of life that lack physical form yet stir the deepest waters of your soul. Whether it's a connection to nature, a profound piece of music, or the embrace of human relationships, spirituality is the tapestry of light and shadow that paints your life with meaning, transcending the mere accumulation of days into an art of living with purpose and fulfillment.

The roots of spiritual sickness

The journey into spiritual discomfort often begins with a subtle departure from the rituals and routines that ground and center your being. When you abandon daily spiritual practices, a disconnection festers, severing the ties to your innermost self. This gap widens without the nurturing acts of meditation, reflective writing, or simple mindfulness that anchor you in the present. The absence of a spiritual regimen sows seeds of emptiness, which, if left unattended, can grow into a pervasive sense of spiritual malaise.

Harboring resentment and withholding forgiveness create burdens that weigh heavily on your soul. Just as physical wounds require care to heal, emotional injuries also need your attention and intention to mend. When you allow grudges to reside within you, they fester, poisoning your inner world and cultivating an environment ripe for spiritual sickness. Narcissism — an excessive focus on oneself at the expense of others — can disrupt the balance of giving and receiving, leading to a spiritually imbalanced life.

The ecosystems we inhabit — our homes, workplaces, social circles — profoundly influence our spiritual well-being. Dwelling in unhealthy environments, where dissent and negativity flourish, crushes the spirit, smothering any spark of serenity and peace. In this context, strained relations are constant stressors that chip away at your spiritual resilience. A breach of personal values — the ideals and morals that define who you aim to be — can lead to an internal conflict, leaving you feeling adrift and morally compromised.

Trauma and unresolved issues are potent roots of spiritual sickness. They're like storms that leave deep scars on the landscape of your psyche, affecting how you perceive and interact with the world around you. When rehearsed repeatedly, negative thought patterns become entrenched in your mind, shaping a reality where hope and positivity struggle to exist. These roots of spiritual sickness, if unaddressed, can immobilize you, trapping you in a cycle of pain and disconnection that undermines the essence of your spirituality.

Consequences of untreated spiritual malady

Neglecting your spiritual health doesn't merely impact your inner peace; it has tangible consequences on your relationships and your ability to recover from past traumatic events. The stress you carry unaddressed can become a weight that hinders your personal growth and strains your connections with those around you, leaving scars far more profound than any physical ailment.

When your spirituality suffers, it's like denying nourishment to a crucial part of your being that is meant to give life and energy to your everyday actions. The symptoms of this malady can manifest as perpetual discomfort, agitation, or the feeling of "white-knuckling" through life — barely holding on instead of thriving. Your ability to handle situations gracefully diminishes, leaving you lacking humility and a self-centered demeanor. These signs indicate a deeper imbalance that, if left unchecked, leads to a life peppered with conflicts and misunderstandings.

Moreover, an untreated spiritual condition results in a feeling of bankruptcy of the soul — a profound disconnection that leaves you grappling with a lack of motivation and purpose. You might find yourself withdrawing into isolation, your mind clouded with distorted thinking and selfishness. In extreme cases, this may even necessitate intervention from others to help you recognize the gravity of the situation. Spirituality, often being a personal and intangible aspect of life, can be the last thing you consider attending to during difficult times, yet it is precisely what requires your focus to foster a foundational change.

REMEMBER

Your journey toward spiritual wellness should regard the roots of spiritual sickness with care to mend the path ahead. The roots often stem from not maintaining a spiritual practice, carrying unresolved burdens, or living in unhealthy environments that do not align with your values. Addressing these issues can illuminate the way to meaningful recovery, helping you rebuild relationships and reduce the emotional and psychological stress disrupting your peace. Cultivating a practice of forgiveness, self-awareness, and active pursuit of things that nurture your spirit are critical steps toward healing and overall emotional resilience.

CONSEQUENCES OF UNTREATED SPIRITUAL MALADY: PATH TO REDEMPTION WITH SAMANTHA

A thread of darkness lurked within Samantha — a shadow that concealed the agony of her spiritual malady. Unseen and often unrecognized, this internal affliction runs deeper than the physical dependence on any substance; it's the profound disconnection from self, others, and life's true essence. It's the void that Samantha tried to fill with the numbing embrace of IV heroin, a desperate attempt to silence the discord within.

Like many before her, the consequences of her untreated spiritual malady manifested as a relentless pursuit of fulfillment through the deceptive solace of drugs. Samantha found herself caught in the vicious cycle of her addiction, which only deepened her spiritual wounds and compounded her existential despair.

Her continuous battles with addiction thrust her into a world of shadows, where hope flickered dimly like a candle in a windstorm. The persistent emptiness, the profound disconnection, and the lack of purpose gnawed at her soul, driving her to seek momentary escape but leading her further into incarceration and desolation.

Yet, within Samantha's story of darkness lies a turning point — a realization that her unaddressed spiritual sickness not only fueled her addiction but was the key to her liberation. The moment she discerned the true nature of her battle, she found the courage to reach for help, to ask for guidance, and to embark on a transformative journey of recovery that would redefine her existence.

Embracing a holistic approach to her healing, Samantha sought to mend the fragmented pieces of her being. Therapy and counseling became her sanctuaries of introspection, where she delved into the mire of her pain and trauma. Support groups provided her with fellowship and understanding — a collective strength to replace the isolation she had known for so long.

It was in these moments of vulnerability that Samantha's true healing began. She discovered the concept known as the Law of

(continued)

(continued)

Attraction, which is the idea that positive or negative thoughts can bring positive or negative experiences into your life. In simple terms, it means that what you focus on mentally and emotionally can shape your reality.

Samantha realized how powerful her thoughts and beliefs could be. She learned to visualize a life free from addiction, speak affirmations that reminded her of her innate worth, and let go of the resistance that kept her tied to her past. Through this practice, she started to reclaim her life and move towards a healthier, more positive future.

Spiritual practices became the bedrock upon which she rebuilt her life. Meditation, gratitude, and nature provided the serenity she craved, while yoga and creative expression became conduits for processing her emotions and releasing her trauma. Through service to others, Samantha found a purpose that transcended her own journey, amplifying her healing by sharing it with the world.

As Samantha pieced back the mosaic of her relationships, she confronted the consequences of her addiction head-on. She approached each bond with humility and truth, restoring trust through consistency and transformation. These relationships, once marred by the effects of her spiritual malady, now blossomed under the light of her newfound authenticity and commitment to growth.

Today, Samantha stands as a testament to the resilience of the human spirit. Her journey from the depths of addiction to a place of empowerment is a narrative that shines with hope for anyone trapped in the grips of spiritual malady. Her story imparts a profound message: Healing is possible, wholeness is attainable, and life, when reclaimed, is a symphony of purpose and joy.

This is not simply a chronicle of her past struggles but an affirmation that every individual has the capacity for renewal and transformation. Once defined by the chains of addiction, Samanatha's life is now a beacon of light — a light that guides others through their darkness, proving that the most profound transformations often stem from the deepest wounds.

Cultivating Spiritual Wellness

Spiritual wellness is not merely an abstract concept; it's a tangible and critical aspect of your recovery that permeates all facets of life. Cultivating your spiritual wellness means consistently nurturing and growing in the areas of your life that bring deeper meaning and connection. It's the antidote to relapse, the balm for frayed relationships, and the boost to self-esteem and confidence desperately needed when life seems bleak. But what does it mean to cultivate spiritual wellness? It's about nurturing the part of you that connects to something larger than yourself — whatever that may be — to thrive, not just survive.

Your journey into spiritual wellness might begin with defining what spirituality means to you. It's personal and unique, ranging from belief in a Higher Power, a set of values, or even the energy of love that binds people together. Embracing this can bring a profound sense of purpose and direction, standing as a beacon when faced with life's challenges. Establishing daily practices —breathing exercises, meditative walks in nature, or engaging in fulfilling hobbies — lays the stepping stones for a resilient and centered life.

Creating a routine that promotes your spiritual health can include simple practices such as prayer, meditation, or contemplative writing, which all work toward grounding you in the present moment. It's also about finding joy and peace in the small things and allowing yourself to be open to experience and growth. Remember, cultivating a spiritual practice is not about achieving perfection but consistently engaging in practices that align with your spirit and enrich your life.

Establishing intimate connections with friends or mentors can also be integral to your spiritual toolkit. By providing a safe space to share and listen, you cultivate an environment where you and your confidant can grow spiritually. Write a letter to the unknown, ask for guidance during quiet moments, or simply share in the silence. These interactions can reveal insights and foster a deep sense of mutual understanding and support on your path to spiritual wellness.

Spiritual values as a power — 12 spiritual principles for long-term recovery

Spiritual principles form the foundation of many successful recovery programs, originating from enduring traditions prioritizing personal growth and self-reflection. These principles are not recent innovations but rather the culmination of centuries-old practices adapted to address the challenges of modern addiction and recovery. Their significance lies in the universal truths they embody — about human nature, the need for community, personal responsibility, and the search for meaning beyond oneself.

Society grapples with the complexities of addiction, and these spiritual principles have become increasingly valuable. They offer a structured approach to overcoming the seemingly insurmountable obstacles posed by substance abuse. Grounded in the practical application of ethical and moral codes, they provide a clear framework for individuals to rebuild their lives, restore their integrity, and maintain long-term sobriety. These principles are embraced for their ability to instill hope, instigate change, and foster resilience; they are crucial in the ongoing quest for a balanced and fulfilling life free from the bonds of addiction.

As we examine the 12 spiritual principles, we'll uncover how each one reinforces the delicate structure of sobriety, providing a comprehensive guide for achieving a more meaningful life.

1. **Honesty:** The journey to sobriety is paved with the stone of honesty. It requires confronting the brutal truth about one's addiction, acknowledging personal flaws, and accepting reality without the distortion of substances. To employ honesty, keep a journal where you can express your thoughts and feelings candidly.

   Example: Jane admits to her support group that she's struggling with cravings rather than pretending to be in control.

2. **Hope:** Hope is the belief that change is possible and recovery can be attained. The light pierces through the darkest hours of withdrawal and doubt. Cultivate hope by surrounding yourself with success stories of recovery and maintaining a vision board that encapsulates your aspirations.

Example: Mark finds hope by attending meetings and listening to the stories of those who have achieved multiple years of sobriety.

3. **Faith:** Faith is trust in a Higher Power, the recovery process, or something else. It is the unwavering conviction that one is not alone in this journey. Practice faith by engaging in daily meditation, focusing on the connection with a power greater than yourself.

   Example: Sarah practices faith by believing that her Higher Power will give her the strength to resist temptation.

4. **Courage:** Courage is the bravery to confront fears, make amends, and change destructive patterns. It involves stepping out of one's comfort zone to achieve growth. Display courage by tackling complex tasks head-on, such as making amends to those you've wronged.

   Example: David uses courage to transform his actions and reconcile with a friend he had harmed during his period of active addiction.

5. **Integrity:** Integrity is the alignment of actions and values. It means living in truth and upholding moral principles. You incorporate integrity into your daily existence by consistently making decisions aligned with your principles, regardless of whether others are observing you.

   Example: Emily practices integrity by refusing to gossip about a co-worker, aligning her behavior with her values of kindness and respect.

6. **Willingness:** Willingness is the readiness to embrace change and follow through with the recovery steps. It's an open-minded approach to new ideas and ways of living. Show willingness by volunteering for service opportunities and being proactive in your recovery plan.

   Example: Carlos shows willingness by accepting a mentor's suggestion to try a new recovery meeting.

7. **Humility:** Humility is acknowledging one's limitations and the openness to learn and grow from others. It's an antidote to ego and arrogance. Practice humility by seeking guidance and accepting that you do not have all the answers.

Example: Lisa embraces humility by asking for help when overwhelmed rather than struggling alone.

8. **Love:** Love is the unconditional acceptance and compassion for oneself and others. It is the force that binds communities and heals wounds. Express love by engaging in acts of kindness and self-care, ensuring love is a daily practice.

   Example: John expresses love by volunteering at a local shelter, offering compassion and service to those in need.

9. **Discipline:** Discipline is the steady practice of recovery activities. It is the commitment to maintain daily routines that support sobriety. Enforce discipline by adhering to a structured schedule that includes time for self-reflection, exercise, and relaxation.

   Example: Anita demonstrates discipline by attending daily meditation sessions despite her busy schedule.

10. **Patience:** Patience is the ability to endure the process of recovery without succumbing to frustration or despair. It involves trusting the pace of one's journey. Practice patience by setting realistic goals and celebrating small victories.

    Example: Tom practices patience by acknowledging that his road to recovery will have ups and downs, and not every day will be easy.

11. **Perseverance:** Perseverance is the steadfast dedication to continue despite challenges and setbacks. It's the commitment to keep moving forward. Fortify perseverance by reminding yourself of how far you've come and the goals you're working toward.

    Example: Danielle perseveres by attending her support group meetings, even after experiencing a relapse, and recommitting to her sobriety.

12. **Service:** Service is the act of giving back to others and the community. It's a way to reinforce one's recovery by supporting others. Engage in service by becoming a sponsor, sharing your experiences, or volunteering in recovery-related activities.

    Example: Aiden finds purpose in service by mentoring newcomers in his recovery program and helping them navigate the early stages of sobriety.

These 12 spiritual principles are the pillars upon which long-term sobriety is built. They are not merely concepts to be understood; instead, they are practices to be woven into your daily life. By living these principles, you can establish a foundation that supports your sobriety and enriches your existence with more profound meaning and connection. As each day dawns, let these values guide you to a brighter, more resilient, and purposeful life.

Embracing a Higher Power

Often embraced within recovery programs, spiritual principles stand as monumental guideposts for achieving and maintaining long-term sobriety. Think of these principles as a potential *power* that looms larger than your self — spiritual tools you can harness to connect with a Higher Power. They represent discipline, hope, faith, courage, honesty, willingness, humility, love, justice, perseverance, spirituality, and service.

Each principle can deeply transform your life by guiding you toward ethical living, self-awareness, and altruism, which transcend mere human strength. As you integrate these principles, they become your steadfast companions on the road to recovery. When combined with acknowledging a Higher Power, as detailed in this chapter, these pillars provide a robust framework that supports sobriety and your entire spiritual journey. Through their application, you acknowledge a force far greater than yourself, a source of unwavering strength and inspiration, helping you navigate the complexities of life with a renewed sense of purpose and serenity.

You might feel hesitant when you hear "Higher Power." Your mind may jump to structured religion or specific deities that don't resonate with your belief system. However, the concept of a Higher Power in the context of recovery and spiritual wellness is much more inclusive and personal. Think of a Higher Power as an expansive energy that transcends individual existence — one that can be found in the profound love we experience, the awe-inspiring beauty of nature, or the steadfast values we hold dear. It connects to the core of your being and provides a larger sense of meaning and direction. It doesn't have to fit into any box; it just needs to feel true and supportive to you.

Accepting a Higher Power into your life is a personal journey where you choose what has meaning for you and how it influences your life. It involves recognizing a supportive force that can guide you through difficult times and comfort you when you're unsure. This step is crucial for spiritual health — vital for staying sober and satisfied with life. Building a relationship with this greater force, whether through quiet reflection, prayer, or being in nature, gives you a practical way to find stability and peace amid daily challenges.

Embracing a Higher Power can be a deeply personal and transformative experience. Here are seven ideas that outline various ways to connect with a Higher Power, each offering a unique approach for each day of the week:

1. Monday — Contemplative meditation:

- Find a quiet space and sit comfortably.
- Begin with deep breaths to center yourself.
- Meditate on the concept of a Higher Power and its presence in your life.
- Allow thoughts and feelings to flow without judgment as you connect with this force.

2. Tuesday — Nature immersion:

- Spend time in a natural setting such as a park, forest, or beach.
- Observe the beauty around you and recognize it as a manifestation of the Higher Power.
- Reflect on the interconnectedness of all things.

3. Wednesday — Scriptural study:

- Choose texts or scriptures that resonate with your understanding of a Higher Power.
- Read and ponder the words, seeking insights and personal revelations.
- Journal your thoughts and feelings about the passages.

4. Thursday — Creative expression:

- Engage in artistic activities such as painting, writing, or playing music.
- Dedicate this act of creation to your Higher Power.
- Reflect on how this process makes you feel connected to a source of inspiration greater than yourself.

5. Friday — Acts of service:

- Perform an act of kindness or service for someone else.
- Do this to honor the Higher Power by serving others.
- At the end of the day, reflect on how service strengthens your relationship with the Higher Power.

6. Saturday — Prayer or affirmation:

- Begin and end your day with a prayer or affirmation acknowledging the Higher Power.
- Repeat this prayer or affirmation throughout the day, especially during challenging moments.
- Notice the feelings of support and comfort that come from this practice.

7. Sunday — Community connection:

- Participate in a community event, workshop, or service that aligns with your spiritual values.
- Engage with others who share your belief in a Higher Power, and draw strength from this collective faith.
- Share experiences and learn from the spiritual insights of others.

By following this schedule, you can immerse yourself in a holistic experience that deepens your connection to a Higher Power and allows you to explore this connection through various dimensions of your life. Each day provides an opportunity for growth and reflection, ultimately contributing to a profound spiritual journey.

For many on the path of recovery, acknowledging a Higher Power can be transformative. It's not about surrendering control but acknowledging that there are elements of life beyond our direct influence that can offer strength and guidance. Whether it's the humbling expanse of the universe, the unconditional love of a pet, or deeply held principles that steer your moral compass, inviting a Higher Power into your life can equip you with a compass to navigate life's challenges. It is a personal testament to the belief that you are part of something bigger, something that can nourish your spirit and fortify your resolve to thrive in sobriety and beyond.

Navigating the journey of recovery or living an alcohol-free life can be rewarding and deeply personal. While traditional recovery programs often reference a "Higher Power," not everyone connects with the concept of God as it's commonly understood. Luckily, the beauty of this journey is that it's customizable; you can define a Higher Power in a way that resonates with you.

A STORY OF HOPE AND FORGIVENESS WITH SALLY

Sally, sober for two decades, had never let the glow of her Higher Power dim — until the unthinkable tore through the fabric of her reality. Her 17-year-old daughter, a bright-eyed soul who mirrored Sally's own strength and had never witnessed the shadow of her mother's past battles with addiction, was stolen from this world by a drunk driver. The irony was a cruel cut, severing Sally's connection to the faith that had been her lifeline.

Her daughter had been a constant by her side in the meeting halls, a silent witness to the collective strength that recovery can build. Once anchored by the 12 principles, Sally's world is now in the abyss of despair.

The principles that had been her safety net morphed into the lifelines tugging at the edges of her grief. She faced each day invoking the spirit of those tenets — discipline to maintain a routine, hope to see through the fog, faith as frayed as it was, and courage to confront the pain.

The day of reckoning came when she had to sit in the courtroom, eyes fixed on the person whose actions had shattered her world. There, amidst the murmurs and palpable tension, the principle of forgiveness approached her like a long-lost friend. She reached out with a trembling hand, grasping it as her daughter would have — firmly and with conviction. Understanding the disease of alcoholism, this person suffered with, as did she.

In that courtroom, Sally whispered the words of forgiveness, not for the person who caused the pain, but for herself to be free from the anchor of bitterness, and right then, something transcendent stirred within her. A warm, almost ethereal sensation filled the void left by her lost connection, and there she felt it — a presence, her Higher Power, returning to her in her moment of unconditional surrender.

She didn't leave the courtroom with her daughter's hand in hers, but she carried the weight of her memory transformed into a new purpose. Sally's Higher Power had not abandoned her; it had been waiting for her to emerge through the principles that had once saved her. Restored to life by this act of grace, Sally understood that her journey hadn't ended — it had been given a new beginning, guided by an unseen but ever-present force and the daughter whose spirit would forever inspire her path of recovery and forgiveness.

Discovering your personal values collage

Here's a simple, non-preachy exercise to help you explore your version of a Higher Power. The Personal Values Collage exercise is inspired by various holistic and self-discovery practices that encourage personal reflection and creativity. The idea is to use expressive tools to explore concepts that are meaningful to an individual, even when they don't subscribe to traditional religious beliefs.

Materials needed:

>> A selection of magazines, images, or access to a printer

>> A large piece of paper or poster board

>> Glue or tape

>> Markers or pens

Steps:

1. **Reflect:** Spend a few moments thinking about the qualities you admire in others or aspire to embody — like kindness, courage, love, or wisdom.

2. **Search and compile:** Look through your materials and find images, words, or quotes representing these qualities. Don't overthink it; trust your instincts.

3. **Assemble your collage:** Arrange the images and words on your paper or poster board. As you place each item, consider how it connects to your personal values and sense of inner strength.

4. **Give it a name:** Once your collage feels complete, consider if a word, phrase, or name captures the essence of your Higher Power. Write it boldly on your collage.

5. **Reflect again:** Look at your collage and consider how this representation can guide and support you. How does it help you feel connected to something larger than yourself?

REMEMBER

Your Higher Power can be an ideal, a set of principles (as discussed above), the best version of yourself, or even the interconnectedness of humanity and the universe. It's a personal touchstone that gives you strength and perspective, particularly in challenging times.

Feel free to return to your collage when you need a reminder or want to add something new. It's a living representation of your evolving understanding of a Higher Power that's uniquely yours.

Embracing a concept of a Higher Power that's meaningful to you can be a source of comfort and strength in your alcohol-free journey. You don't have to fit into any prescribed notions — what matters most is what supports and inspires you.

Practices that promote spiritual health

Cultivating your spiritual health is a deeply personal journey, and the beauty lies in its unique expression for each individual. You don't have to follow a prescribed path or dedicate extensive periods to silent retreats — unless that's where you find your serenity. It's about discovering and nurturing practices that sing to your soul and connect you with a higher energy, be it love, the universe, or your own set of guiding values. Whether through mindful breathing exercises that center your thoughts or the quiet reflection of prayer, these moments of connection are the cornerstones of your spiritual well-being.

By following this grid, you can immerse yourself in a holistic experience that deepens your personal connection to a Higher Power and allows you to explore this connection through various dimensions of your life. Each day provides an opportunity for growth and reflection, ultimately contributing to a profound spiritual journey.

Incorporating these practices into your daily life can be as simple as a morning stretch to the sun or a few silent affirmations before starting your day. Journaling brings you solace, allowing you to pour out your innermost thoughts and connect with your higher self on paper. Or maybe it's the rhythmic movement of a long walk in the park, where the whispers of nature speak to you. No matter how small, every action can be infused with spiritual significance with mindfulness and a heartfelt intention to align with your more profound truths.

Consistency in these practices is key to reaping their full benefits. Just as muscles require regular exercise to maintain strength, your spiritual health flourishes with repeated nurturing. You can set aside a special time and space each day for this purpose, creating a personal sanctuary where you can retreat and refill your spirit. Over time, these practices become sacred rituals, anchoring you in the present and building resilience against life's turbulence. They are less about the specific activity and more about your dedication to fostering inner peace and strength on your journey toward recovery.

Remember, spiritual health is not about perfection — it's about progress. Each step you take, no matter how tentative, is a victory. Whether you're drawn to the soothing practice of contemplative writing or find a spiritual connection in the familiar chords of your favorite song, embrace these activities that resonate with your being. They are your tools for self-empowerment, your allies in the quest for a balanced and fulfilling sober life. So, take a moment today to ask yourself what spiritual practice you can begin or deepen. Your path to spiritual renewal starts with that single, yet powerful, choice.

3

Living (and Loving) a Sober Lifestyle

Learn techniques to resist peer pressure in social settings

Adopt holistic practices for overall well-being

Set and achieve goals that bring purpose and joy to your life

Chapter **7**

Navigating Social Situations

S obriety is a courageous journey that doesn't end with putting down the drink; it extends into every aspect of your daily life, including the complex puzzle of social interactions. Without the crutch of alcohol and other substances, you might find yourself facing the raw reality of social situations, which can be both challenging and empowering. This chapter will guide you through navigating these waters, offering strategies to tackle the awkwardness, develop your social muscles, and find joy in interactions that support your sober life.

In social contexts, especially gatherings or places where alcohol or other substances had once been your social lubricant, you might now experience a heightened sense of awareness about your social anxieties. Rest assured, you are not alone in feeling unwelcomed or anxious at events that revolve around drinking. Whether it's the surprise of discovering alcohol at a social event or the pressure within specific work environments to participate in drinking, these challenges are a normal part of our culture. But there are effective ways to navigate these situations while maintaining your sobriety and dignity.

This chapter teaches you that understanding and applying specific strategies can transform your social life. These include seeking the warmth of a supportive community, finding company in a sober companion, or indulging in non-alcoholic activities — assets that reinforce your sobriety while you navigate social terrains. With the tools discussed in this chapter, socializing can become a nourishing and delightful part of your new sober life.

Socializing in Sobriety: Strategies and Challenges

The transition into living in long-term sobriety brings about a different landscape of socializing — one without the familiar presence of alcohol or other mind-altering substances. It reveals unexpected situations and challenges that test your resilience and commitment. From networking events laden with wine to celebrations where the champagne flows freely, the sober individual often confronts a world that doesn't seem to cater to their lifestyle choices.

Critical strategies for managing this shift focus on creating a supportive social setup. A sober companion can be a tremendous asset in these situations, offering camaraderie and understanding when it feels like no one else can. Meanwhile, engaging in non-alcoholic activities such as joining improv classes, participating in Toastmasters, or spending time at dog parks can be instrumental in building a sober routine that is both fulfilling and socially rewarding.

Acknowledging and embracing social anxiety or awkwardness as a natural part of your growth process is crucial. Professional help can be a vital resource in coping and developing the necessary skills to thrive in social settings while sober. Additionally, aligning with like-minded individuals who value personal growth and new experiences can be comforting and inspiring as you navigate this next chapter in your social life.

REMEMBER

While your sobriety journey may shift your social landscape, it also opens the door to genuine connection and self-discovery. Challenges will inevitably arise as you navigate events and environments steeped in alcohol culture. Still, with a supportive network and a roster of sober activities, each social interaction becomes an opportunity for growth. Embrace your sober identity with confidence, knowing that the strategies you build — finding a sober companion, engaging in new hobbies, and seeking professional guidance — will transform these challenges into stepping stones for a rewarding and resilient sober life.

The mindful sobriety social quest

Mindfully rehearse and fortify your social engagement skills through imaginative and reflective exercises:

Materials needed:

>> A journal or notepad

>> Pen or pencil

>> A timer (a kitchen timer or smartphone will work)

>> A comfortable and quiet spot to sit and think

Instructions:

1. The imagination stage:

- Find a cozy nook where you can relax without interruptions.

- Close your eyes and envision entering a grand party where everyone is in high spirits, and drinks are offered left and right.

2. The social strategy visualization:

- Start the timer for 5 minutes.

- In your mind's eye, visualize a host approaching you with a tray of alcoholic beverages. Mentally rehearse a polite but firm refusal, and see yourself requesting a non-alcoholic alternative with confidence.

- Play this mental script a few times, altering your response to keep it natural and spontaneous.

3. **The conversation gauntlet:**
   - Without opening your eyes, imagine conversing with a total stranger.
   - Challenge yourself to keep the dialogue flowing for another 5 minutes without mentioning alcohol or your sobriety.
   - If you get stuck, think about topics such as travel, music, food, or current events — areas that can spark engaging discussions.

4. **The compliment circuit:**
   - Still, in your visualization, seek out guests who look interesting and imagine paying them a compliment on something other than their appearance, like their energy or an insightful comment they made.
   - Think about how you can use compliments to bridge into deeper conversations.

5. **The art of excuse:**
   - Now, mentally practice a scenario where you need to step away from an uncomfortable conversation or decline an activity that doesn't align with your sobriety.
   - Use your timer to give yourself just two minutes to devise a graceful exit strategy, such as, "I'm so sorry, but I have to make sure and pick up my kids in 20 minutes. . ."

6. **The empathy engine:**
   - Imagine another guest confides in you about their challenges with sobriety or a different personal issue.
   - Reflect on how you'd provide support and understanding without becoming an impromptu therapist.

7. **The reflective wrap-up:**
   - Open your eyes and take a few moments to jot down in your journal key insights, phrases, and strategies you came up with.

- Write down any feelings or discoveries that arose during your mental rehearsal.

8. **Bonus! The laugh track:**

- For a fun twist, think of the most outlandish, silly refusals or conversation topics you might use. This can reduce the perceived gravity of social interactions and add a layer of humor to your preparation.

Regularly engaging in the "the sobriety social quest" trains your brain to handle various social situations with grace, wit, and sobriety. Plus, infusing your humor and playful scenarios makes the exercise fun and light-hearted; you can use it with many different scenarios. The more you mentally rehearse, the more equipped and relaxed you'll feel when it's time to shine in a real-world social setting — all while embracing your alcohol-free lifestyle!

Developing social skills in recovery

As you embrace long-term recovery, developing new social skills is akin to learning a language — you'll start with basics and then work your way up to fluency. When alcohol no longer takes up space in your social repertoire, you need to fill that vacancy with sober skills that help you connect with others. Socialization in recovery can be nurtured in sober-friendly environments, such as game nights, barbecues, or other activities where the focus isn't on drinking but on shared experiences instead.

Sober bars are a trend that recognizes the need for inclusive social settings. Instead of feeling the pressure to drink, you can enjoy a space where your choice to stay sober is not just accepted but celebrated. Sobriety in a sales environment, for instance, can be particularly trying, but being transparent about your recovery can eliminate peer pressure and potentially inspire others as well.

Setting boundaries is critical to further developing social adept-ness. This involves assertiveness in educating others about your sobriety and understanding your audience when sharing your recovery story. Create a space where you feel comfortable and respected and where you can form genuine connections without the presence of alcohol. Cultivate your skills, choose your settings wisely, and watch your social sphere blossom.

Creating a social activity tracker

Embarking on your recovery journey introduces the necessity to hone social skills that may have been atrophied by past alcohol use. Learning and practicing ways of connecting with people who don't rely on substances is essential. The environments you socialize in play a significant role in this learning process. Incorporating a social activity tracker into your alcohol-free journey can be an enlightening and motivating experience. A social activity tracker serves as a personalized log where you can record the various sober activities you engage in, along with your emotional responses and the quality of social interactions you experience. By monitoring these aspects over time, you can identify which activities uplift your mood, enrich your social life, and contribute most positively to your overall well-being.

Here's how to set up and use your social activity tracker:

1. **Create your tracker:** Choose a format that works best for you. This could be a digital spreadsheet, a handwritten journal, or a printable template. Your tracker should have columns or sections for:

   - **Date and time:** When did the activity occur?
   - **Activity description:** What did you do? Be specific.
   - **People involved:** Who did you interact with?
   - **Duration:** How long did the activity last?
   - **Mood before activity (1-10):** Rate your mood before starting the activity.
   - **Mood after activity (1-10):** Rate your mood immediately after the activity.
   - **Social connection (1-10):** Rate your sense of connection with others during the activity.
   - **Notes:** Write down your thoughts or feelings about the activity.

2. **Engage in activities:** Start participating in sober activities that interest you. Approach each activity with an open mind.

3. **Record and reflect:** After each social outing or event, take a moment to fill in your tracker. Be honest with your ratings and notes – this is for your eyes only.

4. **Review periodically:** Set aside time each week or month to review your tracker. Look for patterns:

- Which activities consistently improve your mood?

- Which events lead to the highest sense of social connection?

- Are there any activities that don't have the positive impact you expected?

- Based on your reflections, are there new activities you'd like to try?

5. **Adjust and explore:** Based on your observations, make adjustments to your social activity choices. Explore new activities that have the potential to score high on mood and social connection.

Table 7-1 shows a sample social activity tracker entry.

TABLE 7-1 **Sample Social Activity Tracker**

Date	Activity	People Involved	Duration	Mood Before	Mood After	Social Connection	Notes
12-Apr-23	Pottery Class	Classmates, Instructor	2 Hours	6	8	7	Felt relaxed shaping clay. Enjoyed laughter with the group.

TIP

Maintaining your social activity tracker creates a tangible record of how your alcohol-free life unfolds. It's a powerful tool for recognizing the rewarding aspects of sobriety and steering your social life in a direction that consistently brings you joy and fulfillment. This proactive approach can solidify your commitment to an alcohol-free lifestyle and remind you of the vibrant life you're building, one activity at a time.

Addressing social anxiety and awkwardness

Dealing with social anxiety and discomfort in sobriety isn't just about bravery — it's about strategy. It may require stepping out of your comfort zone and embracing the initial awkwardness of social growth. Socializing may initially amplify your uncertainties, making events like improv classes or Toastmasters seem daunting, but these situations are the best opportunities for personal evolution.

A supportive community can be an essential touchstone on your journey. When you're part of a group that shares similar sobriety goals, it's easier to work through your social anxiety together. And if needed, seeking professional help can be a significant step toward overcoming these barriers. It's about recognizing your needs, being proactive in getting the proper support, and permitting yourself to be authentically you — embracing your awkward moments.

Selecting sober-friendly environments is not just about comfort but also about thriving in your sober life. From enjoying the quiet companionship of a dog park to laughing genuinely with newfound friends at a comedy night, these settings foster genuine and enriching interactions. As you frequent these spaces and engage with like-minded individuals, you will find that your social anxiety and awkwardness diminish, leaving you with more robust connections and a more confident self.

The following exercise will help you steady yourself when social anxiety reveals itself. Here, you'll create a social scavenger hunt:

Objective:

Gradually expose yourself to social environments in a structured and goal-oriented way to help manage social anxiety and build confidence in social settings.

Instructions:

1. **Create list:** Start by listing social environments that make you slightly anxious but are manageable — think coffee shops, bookstores, community events, or local meetups related to your hobbies or interests.

2. **Create quests:** Create a "quest" for each location that involves interacting with others. This could be as simple as asking a barista for a coffee recommendation or joining a group at a meetup and asking what brought them there.

3. **Set intentions:** Set an intention before embarking on each quest. It could be to learn something new about a person, to share a bit about your sobriety journey, or simply to enjoy a conversation without judgment.

4. **Increase the difficulty gradually:** Gradually increase the difficulty of your quests. After you're comfortable in one setting, move on to one that provides a bit more challenge, like attending a sober potluck or a recovery meeting.

5. **Reflect:** After each interaction, take a moment to reflect. Write down what went well, what you learned, and how you felt before, during, and after the interaction.

6. **Celebrate:** Celebrate your progress, no matter how small. Acknowledging your bravery and the steps you're taking is paramount.

7. **Track your progress:** Keep a journal or a log on your phone to track your progress. Note the date, the place, the quest, your pre-quest feelings, and post-quest reflections. Observing your growth over time can be incredibly encouraging.

8. **Seek professional support:** If you find that your anxiety is more than just jitters, consider seeking the help of a therapist to develop personalized strategies for managing social anxiety.

TIP

Pair up with a fellow sober friend looking to expand their social skills. For support, tackle the social scavenger hunt together!

Embarking on these social quests can help you turn what once felt like a daunting odyssey into an enjoyable time of connection and growth. Discover the treasures of interpersonal connection; sober relations, outings, and connections are not to be missed!

Choosing sober-friendly social settings

Selecting environments that align with your lifestyle is crucial when navigating the social scene in sobriety. Sober-friendly settings provide a haven where you can socialize without the temptation or pressure of alcohol. From creativity-fueled events like painting classes to the camaraderie of sports leagues, these venues offer many options that support your sober journey.

The environments you choose should encourage sobriety and the joy of social interaction. Examples like game nights and barbecues within sober communities are prime opportunities to connect with others while nurturing your recovery. In your quest to find these settings, don't hesitate to suggest alternatives to alcohol-focused gatherings. Be the one to propose a hike, a game of bowling, or a local community event where alcohol is not the center of attraction. As you do, you'll discover a world of engaging activities offering rich social experiences and catering to your sober lifestyle while educating others about the vast possibilities of sober fun.

Creating a plan B activity tracker

Keep a trusty "sober plan B" up your sleeve. Whether it's suggesting a coffee shop jazz night instead of a bar crawl or having a mocktail menu in mind at a dinner party, be the maestro of your social life by planning alternatives that align with your sobriety. By doing so, you're not just sidestepping the alcohol; you're crafting memorable, authentic experiences with the people you care about — sans the buzz.

Materials needed:

» A notebook or sheet of paper

» A pen or pencil

» Sticky notes (optional)

1. **Set up your tracker:** At the top of a new page in your notebook, write "Plan B Activity Tracker."

2. **Create columns:** Draw three columns labeled "Activity," "Why It's Appealing," and "Preparation Needed."

3. **Brainstorm activities:** In the "Activity" column, list all the sober-friendly activities you enjoy or want to try, such as going to the movies, attending a yoga class, or taking a nature walk.

4. **Explore your interests:** In the "Why It's Appealing" column, write a short note explaining why each activity attracts you. This could be anything from "relaxing," "energizing," or "allows me to meet new people."

5. **Plan ahead:** In the "Preparation Needed" column, jot down any arrangements needed for each activity, such as booking tickets, inviting a friend, or packing a bag.

6. **Use your tracker:** Use this advice for making the most of your tracker:

» **Plan ahead:** Review your tracker at the beginning of each week and decide which activities you'd like to do that week. Schedule them in your calendar.

» **Keep your list handy:** Keep your list handy (physically or on your phone) to quickly pick a Plan B activity if you're ever in a pinch.

» **Reflect and revise:** After participating in an activity, take a moment to note what you enjoyed about it. If it didn't meet your expectations, consider tweaking it for next time or replacing it with something else.

» **Stick to it:** If you use sticky notes, you can place them in your planner or on your fridge as colorful reminders of the fun activities you have planned.

Dealing with Peer Pressure and External Expectations

Living in the world of sobriety can often feel like stepping into a new social landscape. You find yourself navigating unfamiliar territories where the usual markers — bars, parties brimming with alcohol, and gatherings centered on drinking — no longer serve as landmarks. Instead, you're tasked with charting a path that aligns with your sobriety commitment, which may expose you to peer pressure and external expectations. Yet, this very journey can redefine your social experiences and enhance your recovery.

A long, sober lifestyle doesn't require you to forsake social engagements but to approach them with a renewed mindset. It's about rediscovering the joy in connections not lubricated by alcohol, cultivating friendships that support your sober journey, and learning to engage in activities that entertain without the need for substances. Sobriety hands you the opportunity to sculpt a social life that is fulfilling and nurturing to your new way of life. Embrace it as a chance to build meaningful relationships and experiences grounded in authenticity.

REMEMBER

Facing peer pressure and external expectations is part of the landscape when you decide to live a long, sober life. But it's important to stay true to your commitment to sobriety. This isn't about missing out on social events; it's about experiencing them differently and finding joy in authentic connections not defined by alcohol. Your recovery allows you to craft a social life that aligns with your values and supports your well-being. Embrace this opportunity to forge meaningful relationships and create fulfilling experiences on your terms.

Assertiveness in saying "no" to substance use

Envision a scenario at a bustling bar or a celebratory event where you're offered a drink. How do you respond? Assertiveness is your ally in these moments. It's not aggressive to state your non-participation in alcohol consumption; it is a strong, respectful way to honor your sobriety. It's about saying no without justification, guilt, or apprehension. Remember, you owe no one an explanation for your decision. A simple "No, thank you" can be a complete sentence.

Drawing from the increasing popularity of sober bars, you can see how societal views are evolving. Many are choosing to ditch alcohol for healthier lifestyles, creating a trend that supports sobriety. In work environments with a heavy emphasis on drinking, like sales, it's important to hold your ground firmly. Living in recovery is about being transparent about your choices, which, in turn, reduces peer pressure. Assertiveness helps to assert your preference for non-alcoholic drinks and shifts the night from a drinking culture to one of connection and camaraderie.

Being assertive might mean preparing an exit strategy for uncomfortable situations or having a sober companion by your side for support. Recognizing scenarios where you might face peer pressure and coming equipped with strategies is crucial. The goal is to identify and utilize assertive communication, such as clearly stating your preference, using eye contact, and maintaining a courteous yet firm tone. It's quite possible that by doing so, you may become an inspiration for others who are silently wishing to escape the cycle of substance use.

TIP

When you are offered a drink, a firm yet polite "No, thank you" is all you need to say. Confidence is essential, so practice and support your response with assertive body language, such as maintaining eye contact. If you're pressed, repeat your answer firmly — consistency shows conviction. Have a buddy who respects your sobriety for support or an exit strategy if the environment becomes too challenging. Remember, your choice not to drink and live in recovery is valid and requires no explanation. Stay true to your reasons, and take pride in your sobriety.

Setting boundaries with friends and family

In the dance of social interactions, knowing when to step forward and when to step back is crucial, especially when dealing with loved ones. Setting boundaries with friends and family is not about pushing people away; it's about safeguarding your sobriety. It's teaching others how to treat you by clearly outlining what is acceptable in your interactions. Doing so ensures your social environment is conducive to your recovery.

TOAST TO A NEW CHAPTER: FATHERHOOD, FOCUS, AND THE SOBER LIFE WITH CALLUM

My name is Callum, and ever since the divorce papers were inked, life has taken on a sharper focus. I'm a dad first, a sales manager second, and somewhere down that list, a guy rediscovering life sober. It's been quite the journey, and every day I wake up without a hangover feels like a little victory — a win for me and a promise kept to my two amazing kids.

I remember the first time I confidently turned down a drink. I was at one of those expensive corporate mixers where the clinking of glasses was the night's soundtrack. An old colleague slid a drink across the bar to me, his eyes all but chanting, "Come on, just one." I locked eyes with him, offered a grin that meant business, and said, "No thanks, I'm good." It felt like I was taking a stand, not just against the drink, but for myself and the life I was building.

Now, the soccer games with my kids? They're pure joy. I cheer louder and run faster when we play tag; every chuckle from them is music I wouldn't trade for anything. My daughter's impromptu performances in the living room and my son's delighted squeal when he figures out a new puzzle — they're vivid, real, and mine to treasure.

My ex-wife, well, she's even seen the difference. We're navigating this co-parenting journey with a newfound respect, and I can tell it's made all the difference for our kids. They deserve stability and a father they can count on.

Sure, being the sober one among a sea of drinkers can feel like you're navigating a minefield. But I've learned the power of a polite but firm "no." And if things start to feel a bit too wobbly for my liking, I've got my exit strategy — a quick text to check in on the kids that doubles as my cue to slip out.

In the end, I don't need to shout from the rooftops that I'm living sober. The proof is in the quiet moments, the small wins, and the significant milestones with my children. I show up for them daily with clear eyes and a whole heart.

> And if, along the way, I inspire someone else to rethink their dance with the bottle, well, then that's all the better. Because from where I stand — in the shoes of a father, a professional, a friend, and a man who's made peace with his past — life is more prosperous this side of sobriety, and I wouldn't have it any other way.

TIP

These boundaries can range from asking friends not to drink around you to selecting social gatherings that align with your sobriety goals. If events at restaurants and pubs are a typical invitation, suggest alternative venues or activities where alcohol is not the main focus. Express your preference for places like meeting at a museum social or gatherings within sober communities, where you can connect without the presence of alcohol. Upholding such boundaries reinforces your commitment to recovery and gently guides your loved ones to support you meaningfully.

Sometimes, the most challenging part can be talking about your sobriety journey with those closest to you. Building a supportive social network begins with being open and forthcoming about your needs. This includes educating your friends and family about why sobriety is important to you and how they can help. At the end of the day, fostering healthy friendships — relationships that respect your boundaries and support your choices — will contribute greatly to the richness of your social life in sobriety.

TIP

It's essential to communicate your needs directly to those you are with to ensure your relationships support your recovery journey. Let your loved ones know you prefer gatherings where alcohol isn't the main attraction, and suggest specific alternatives. Clear communication about why sobriety matters to you and how they can help is key to building a network that respects your boundaries. Healthy relationships that honor your choices are vital to a fulfilling, alcohol-free social life.

Educating others about your sobriety

While you're not responsible for how others react to your sobriety, you can shape their understanding. Educating others about your sobriety is a way to advocate for yourself and demystify the sober lifestyle. It starts with the realization that not everyone knows how to interact with someone who has chosen a life free from alcohol. You can inform their perspective by sharing your story, but knowing your audience is essential.

When sharing your sobriety journey, consider what you're comfortable disclosing and to whom. Establish a narrative that feels true to you and grants insight without delving into details you'd rather keep private. Whether it's engaging in non-alcoholic activities such as improv classes, Toastmasters, or dog parks, you can show rather than just tell, offering first-hand experiences of how joyous and fulfilling a sober life can be.

Educating others also means being a role model for assertive living. Demonstrating to peers and loved ones how to set boundaries without alienation can also empower them. Returning to the education theme, it's also about knowing when to say enough — is there genuine interest, or has the topic run its course? Maintain your dignity and grace throughout, respecting your story and the people you share it with. Through your actions and openness, you may inspire others and highlight that sobriety is not just a choice — it's a rewarding way of life.

REMEMBER

In guiding others to understand your sobriety, you are crafting an essential narrative that fosters support and respect for your journey. It's important to share your story with dignity and selectiveness, balancing personal insight and privacy. Your experiences and your example set the stage for a respectful, engaging dialogue that can inspire and enlighten those around you.

Creating a Supportive Social Network

Sober living introduces a new set of challenges regarding social interactions. You may find yourself in the center of unexpected situations where alcohol plays a starring role, and the spotlight on your sobriety might feel intense. Confidently navigating this maze starts with understanding that you're not alone in these feelings — and that there's a path through it.

Building a supportive social network is a cornerstone of successful sobriety. Equipping yourself with the right strategies to foster healthy friendships, engage in sober social activities, and connect with like-minded individuals sets a strong foundation. You'll find that with a reliable and understanding group by your side, scenarios that may have once caused unease can be met with a new sense of ease and control.

Let's explore the pathways to developing a social network that respects and uplifts your recovery. Standing firm in your sobriety doesn't have to cost your social life; instead, it's an opportunity to redefine it in ways that align with your values and newfound freedom.

The journey through sobriety doesn't mean your journey alone. A supportive social network is vital in maintaining your sober lifestyle. This network serves as the bulwark against the pressures of socializing in traditionally alcohol-dominated settings and provides refuge when navigating the choppy waters of social engagements. It's about surrounding yourself with people who respect your choices and are there to back you when you're faced with unexpected alcohol-related situations.

TIP

To build a social life in harmony with your sobriety, actively seek out and nurture relationships with individuals and groups who respect your alcohol-free journey. Prioritize engaging in social activities that don't revolve around drinking, such as attending community events, faith-based activities, workshops, or sporting events. Remember, the strength of your social network is not in numbers but in the quality of understanding and support it offers. Keep an eye out for those with similar values and embrace the opportunity to redefine your social circle to enrich your sober lifestyle.

Fostering healthy friendships in sobriety

Building and maintaining healthy friendships is crucial within the refuge of sobriety. These relationships should support your commitment to staying sober rather than compromise it. Codependency should be avoided, and boundaries must be respected. You need friends who not only uphold your decision to be sober but also actively contribute to your life in positive ways. Engaging with a sober community or attending non-alcoholic activities, from improv classes to dog parks, are excellent ways to foster such friendships.

Healthy friendships in sobriety can be rewarding. They provide a support system that helps you through the awkwardness of social anxiety and can significantly ease the process of attending events at restaurants or pubs. Being open about your sobriety is essential, as transparency is the key to eliminating peer pressure and attracting like-minded individuals into your circle.

TIP

When cultivating friendships on your sober journey, seek out individuals who energize and encourage your alcohol-free lifestyle. Prioritize creating a circle of friends who respect your boundaries and are actively involved in alcohol-free environments and hobbies. Openness about your sobriety can serve as a beacon, attracting those on a similar path or supportive allies. Remember, the healthiest friendships in sobriety add to your life without shaking the foundations of your commitment.

Engaging in sober social activities

Sober social activities play a pivotal role in facilitating camaraderie and enjoyment without relying on alcohol. They offer an alternative to traditional alcohol-centric gatherings, allowing you to socialize and connect without compromising your sobriety. Activities such as bowling, comedy nights, dances, hiking, cooking clubs, poetry nights, volunteer work, and mocktail events ensure ample opportunities to interact in settings that prioritize sobriety.

Such activities can significantly enrich your social life by providing diverse experiences focusing on the event itself, not alcohol consumption. For instance, enjoying a game of pickleball or a vegan homemade meal with other vegans or a faith-based book club highlights how recreation can be equally, if not more, fulfilling when it's not shrouded in inebriation. Moreover, the increasing popularity of sober bars exemplifies society's growing embrace of non-alcoholic environments, making it easier to maintain your social life without having to explain or defend your sobriety.

On your vibrant sobriety journey, a whole world of social pleasures is waiting to be discovered that don't require a toast to enjoy. Following is a curated sober social activities list brimming with ideas that aren't just alternatives to alcohol-infused gatherings but experiences that enrich your life and connections. These activities offer diverse options that cater to a wide range of interests, fostering a sense of belonging, excitement, and personal growth. Dive into this list of activities and watch your social calendar bloom with possibilities that affirm the joys of your alcohol-free lifestyle.

Following is a list of sober social activities:

>> Host a game night with various board games and puzzles for a fun and competitive evening.

>> Organize a group to experience the thrill and teamwork of escape rooms.

>> Plan hiking trips or leisurely nature walks in local parks to breathe in fresh air and tranquility.

>> Start a book club focusing on genres that feed the soul, such as personal growth or recovery narratives.

>> Attend or host a sober potluck dinner, where each dish has a story and a unique flavor.

>> Participate in community volunteer work to make a difference and meet others with philanthropic passions.

>> Join a sports league or group fitness classes to boost your health while building team spirit.

>> Explore local museums, galleries, or art exhibits to immerse yourself in culture and inspiration.

>> Create a faith-based book club where you invite writers and authors to discuss your faith.

>> Enroll in a cooking class or workshop to spice up your culinary skills and share delicious creations.

>> Engage in meditation groups or yoga sessions for inner peace and community connection.

>> Attend non-alcoholic music or dance events to feel the rhythm of life without any liquid interference.

>> Try out a new hobby like pottery, painting, or crafting, and let your creativity soar.

- » Plan a sober beach or park day with activities like volleyball, frisbee, or simply soaking in the sun.
- » Set up a movie or documentary night with a curated selection of thought-provoking films.
- » Take part in language learning groups to converse and connect in different tongues.
- » Organize a themed costume party where imagination and attire take center stage.
- » Join a community garden to cultivate plants and friendships in equal measure.
- » Participate in live theater or open mic nights to witness the spontaneous magic of performance.
- » Take up photography and explore your surroundings through the lens of your camera.
- » Join a DIY workshop to learn new crafts like woodworking, knitting, or home decorating.
- » Sign up for a charity run or walkathon, embracing fitness for a good cause.

This list demonstrates that a sober life need not be a social sentence to boredom or isolation. On the contrary, it can be the catalyst for a rich, vibrant social life filled with activities that nourish the soul and foster genuine connections. So, go ahead, mix and match from this list, or use it as a springboard for your own creative ideas. Each activity you choose is another step toward a fulfilling life where every laugh, every discovery, and every triumph is experienced with a clear mind and an open heart. Have fun!

FROM SOLITUDE TO SOCIAL BUTTERFLY WITH SUE

If you had told me ten years ago that I'd be where I am now, I would've shrugged it off. Back then, my social circle was as compact as it could get — just me and my two dogs padding through the concrete jungle of Chicago.

But here I am, a decade into my sobriety, and let me tell you, it's been quite the journey. I used to relish in my solitude, a shield against a world that seemed so drenched in alcohol at every turn. Yet, as I embraced my sober life, I discovered a craving for something more — genuine connections and a tribe that understood the rhythm of my new heartbeat.

How did I go from a loner to a social butterfly, you ask? Well, sober social activities were my golden ticket. I dipped my toes into everything the city had to offer — bowling leagues where strikes and spares were more intoxicating than any drink, comedy nights that had me laughing until my sides hurt, dance classes where the music filled my spirit, and hiking groups that scaled urban jungles and quiet trails alike.

I found camaraderie in cooking clubs, where the sizzle of a pan was our soundtrack, and poetry nights, where words woven in the air stitched us closer together. I even rolled up my sleeves and got involved in volunteer work, where the warmth of helping others became my favorite buzz.

Do you know what surprised me the most? It was the variety and sheer number of people I met who were either on their own sober journeys or just didn't care much for drinking. I didn't need to explain or defend my alcohol-free life; we were all just there to enjoy the moment.

And then there were the sober bars — oh, what a treat! Imagine walking into a bar, ordering a mocktail, and simply chatting away without that old, familiar pressure. It was liberating, and it was in these spots I found some of my closest friends.

With each new experience, my once-small world expanded. I surrounded myself with amazing people who respected my choice and cheered it on. They became my extended family, the ones who understood that joy doesn't come from a bottle — it comes from shared experiences, genuine laughter, and the kind of support that doesn't waver when the night ends.

So, from a former loner with two dogs to the life of the party — sober style — I've woven together this social life that continues to evolve in ways I never imagined. And it all started with the simple choice to live freely, authentically, and joyfully . . . without alcohol.

Building a community of like-minded individuals

When you surround yourself with a community of like-minded individuals, you strengthen your resolve and commitment to sobriety. It's about finding people who are not only sober but committed to personal growth and new experiences. Such communities offer a sense of solidarity and empowerment, reminding you that your sober journey is shared and supported.

Joining groups that resonate with your interests is beneficial. Whether it's participating in a community service project or engaging in a physical fitness class, the interactions you build can be profoundly supportive. This commitment to shared growth fosters a network that isn't just about staying sober but rather evolving and thriving together in sobriety. Together, you'll celebrate milestones, overcome challenges, and enjoy life's activities within a framework that supports and cherishes your sobriety.

REMEMBER

By cultivating a community of like-minded individuals, you're not just maintaining your sobriety but actively enriching your life. Seek out and embrace those who share your commitment to an alcohol-free life and your enthusiasm for personal growth and new experiences. This collective energy will bolster your journey and allow you all to thrive together, creating a powerful synergy of support, empowerment, and shared joy in sobriety's many gifts.

As our exploration of social navigation in sobriety concludes, let's crystallize what you've learned. With its unique challenges, sobriety reshapes your social interactions into something more authentic and rewarding. This chapter equipped you with tools to tackle those moments of awkwardness, fortify your assertiveness, and revel in the joy of connections that rise above the influence of alcohol.

Remember, every event is an opportunity to redefine what socializing means to you. Peer pressure and external expectations will surface but merely echo a past lifestyle. Assertiveness is not just a defense against offers of a drink; it's an affirmation of your commitment to a healthier, more present life.

The strategies discussed here are your compass — pointing you toward supportive communities, sober-friendly activities, and the empowerment to engage with the world on fresh terms. It's about setting boundaries, respecting your journey and fostering relationships celebrating your recovery.

Hold these strategies close as you step into the world committed to long-term sobriety. Use them to navigate through each social setting with confidence and grace. Know that your sobriety is not a limitation but a liberation from the ties that once bound you. Each interaction is a step toward a richer, fuller existence — one you navigate with clarity, purpose, and unwavering commitment to your well-being.

With a new perspective and a set of skills, curate a social life that complements your sobriety. Your journey may inspire others and, collectively, shift the culture toward one where sobriety isn't just accepted — it's respected, embraced, and celebrated.

Chapter 8

Embracing Mental, Physical, and Emotional Well-Being

When you choose to live an alcohol-free life, it's not just about saying "no" to a drink; it's about saying "yes" to a healthier, more vibrant you. Your well-being is at the heart of this life-changing decision. It's about nurturing your body, mind, and spirit to build a life that's not just about surviving without alcohol but thriving in every sense of the word. Understanding your needs and how to care for yourself is the first step toward resilience and happiness in your new life.

In this chapter, you'll discover the tools and strategies for building a fulfilling, alcohol-free life. Through the different sections, we'll explore how to nourish your mental, emotional, and physical health, all interconnected in this beautiful dance of well-being. Let's dive into some of the key takeaways you can expect.

Nurturing Mental Wellness in Sobriety

Sobriety is a journey that entails much more than letting go of alcohol or substances; it embodies the pursuit of holistic well-being, harmonizing the mind, body, and spirit. To nurture your mental wellness while embarking on this path, envision your sobriety as a multifaceted approach, intertwining the absence of alcoholism with nourishing routines that support your overall health. Immerse yourself in a lifestyle that includes a balanced diet rich in nutrients, regular physical activity that energizes your body, and the cultivation of authentic friendships that bring joy and meaning into your life. As you weave these elements together, you lay the foundation for a resilient mental state.

Stepping into the realm of emotional honesty, allow yourself the vulnerability to feel deeply and navigate your emotions without the camouflage of substances. This truthfulness with yourself is a liberating stepping stone in the healing process, one that catalyzes personal growth and fortifies your mental wellness. Sometimes, the pursuit of equilibrium dictates that you step back and take a "mental health day" for self-care and reflection. Far from being selfish, such reprieves are strategic pauses that recharge your capacity to face life's demands, reinforcing your dedication to a sober and balanced life.

In the daily hustle, it's easy to lose sight of the delicate interplay between your emotional and mental states. Mindfulness and meditation are your allies, serving as tools to center your thoughts and foster inner peace. As you cultivate these practices, you anchor yourself in the present moment, warding off the anxious shadows of the past and the uncertainty of the future. These practices, along with healthy coping mechanisms, become your shield against the turbulence of stress and anxiety. Incorporating mindfulness into your routine is not merely a trend; it is a transformative practice that enhances your emotional resilience and supports your journey to lasting sobriety.

Understanding the brain on sobriety

Navigating the world of long-term sobriety isn't just about willpower and good intentions. Scientists have discovered that addiction is deeply rooted in the brain's intricate chemistry and its response to pleasurable stimuli. The neuroscience of addiction is a topic that connects the dots between behavior and brain activity, shedding light on why saying "no" to alcohol isn't as simple as it seems.

When we talk about the neuroscience of addiction, dopamine often takes center stage. It's like the brain's own brand of internal confetti, released to celebrate moments of pleasure and reinforce behaviors necessary for survival, such as eating and reproduction. However, alcohol and other drugs hijack this system, artificially inflating the party to extraordinary levels.

In the brain, dopamine functions as a reward signal that is naturally released following activities experienced as positive or pleasurable. This is an integral part of the brain's reward system, reinforcing behaviors beneficial for survival and well-being. However, alcohol can significantly disrupt this delicate balance. It causes an excessive release of dopamine, rewarding behaviors that are not necessarily good for you. This surge and subsequent overstimulation of the brain's reward pathways can lead to the development of addictive behaviors, as the system begins to associate alcohol consumption with a strong, rewarding sensation, thus overriding the natural order of reward processing.

Over time, consistent alcohol or substance use can lead to alterations in both the structure and the functionality of the brain. Research has revealed that individuals struggling with addiction often exhibit decreased activity in the prefrontal cortex, a critical region for decision-making and impulse control. This reduced activity undermines your ability to resist the urge to drink or use, making it more challenging to abstain from that substance or behavior. This impairment in your prefrontal cortex is a significant neurological consequence of addiction, which can hinder the process of making healthy choices and exercising self-discipline.

Serotonin is an essential neurotransmitter that plays a crucial role in regulating your mood in the brain. When alcohol is abused, it can interfere with serotonin production and regulation, leading to mood disturbances. These alterations in mood can exacerbate the cycle of addiction, as you may turn to alcohol in an attempt to self-medicate and restore your sense of well-being. Therefore, a serotonin deficiency from alcohol use can contribute to a continuous pattern of drinking as a means to alleviate your emotional dysregulation and maintain a semblance of mood stability.

However, as the brain is remarkably adaptable and capable of learning, sobriety can lead to a process known as neuroplasticity, where your brain begins to repair and rewire itself. Engaging in sober activities and treatment can help to fortify your prefrontal cortex, akin to the teacher regaining control of the classroom. New, healthy habits can re-establish normal dopamine function so your brain can once again distribute those gold stars for truly beneficial behaviors.

Understanding the neuroscience behind addiction can empower you on your journey to sobriety. It's not just about abstaining from alcohol; it's about retraining your brain, reshaping your environment, and redefining your life in a way that supports your best self. It's like turning that chaotic classroom back into a place of learning and growth, where every day is an opportunity to earn those gold stars for the right reasons.

REMEMBER

Recovery isn't a solo journey — it's a communal effort, and science is an ally. By combining evidence-based treatments, nutrition, and lifestyle changes, you can work toward a brain environment that supports long-lasting sobriety. It's not just a detox for the body but a rejuvenating process for the brain, where every alcohol-free day is a step toward a healthier, happier mind.

Mindfulness and meditation practices

Embracing mindfulness and meditation can guide you into living more presently and less reactively, allowing you to meet life's events with equanimity. These practices offer stillness for your overactive mind, where the hustle of daily life fades into the background, giving you a space to breathe and center yourself.

Meditation is a practice where you use a technique — such as deep breathing or focusing the mind on a particular object, thought, or activity — to train attention and awareness and achieve a mentally clear, emotionally calm, and stable state. It has been practiced for thousands of years to deepen understanding of life's sacred and mystical forces. Nowadays, meditation is commonly used for stress reduction and relaxation. Science has shown that meditating can have numerous benefits for both the mind and body, including reducing stress, improving concentration, enhancing self-awareness, and promoting a better overall quality of life. From a neuroscientific perspective, several brain regions are implicated in the practice of meditation and its effects on the brain. These regions include:

>> The prefrontal cortex is associated with higher-order brain functions such as awareness, concentration, decision-making, and cognitive flexibility.

>> The anterior cingulate cortex is involved in sustaining attention, monitoring conflicts, and managing emotional responses.

>> The hippocampus plays a significant role in memory formation, memory retention, and emotional regulation.

>> The insula contributes to the body's ability to monitor its internal state and supports self-awareness and emotional experience.

>> The amygdala is related to processing emotions, particularly those related to stress and anxiety.

Regular meditation can actually change the structure of your brain in positive ways. It can make parts of your brain thicker, such as the prefrontal cortex (which is involved in decision-making) and the insula (which helps you understand your own emotions). This suggests that meditation can help your brain adapt and grow.

Changes in the brain can have profound effects on an individual's capacity for self-regulation, resilience to stress, and overall mental well-being. The evidence-based benefits of meditation reflect its potential as a valuable component of a healthy, balanced lifestyle, including in the context of recovery from substance use disorders.

By integrating regular meditation sessions into your routine, you can create an anchor in your day — a moment of respite where clarity and calm become tools to navigate the challenges of sobriety. With each meditation session, you crafting a peaceful mindset that fortifies your mental wellness, supporting your journey to a healthier and more grounded version of yourself.

REMEMBER

Meditation is much more than sitting silently with your legs crossed. It's a journey to the inner workings of your mind, a way to fine-tune your awareness, and a method to achieve a sense of inner peace amidst life's storms. Regular meditation can profoundly sculpt your brain, enhancing regions that sharpen your focus, soothe your emotional seas, and strengthen your memory.

Mindfulness

Mindfulness, the *practice* of maintaining a moment-by-moment awareness of our thoughts, emotions, bodily sensations, and surrounding environment, has roots in Buddhist meditation. The concept was popularized in the West by Jon Kabat-Zinn, an American professor emeritus of medicine. He created the Stress Reduction Clinic and the Center for Mindfulness in Medicine, Health Care, and Society at the University of Massachusetts Medical School. His pioneering work has significantly influenced the integration of mindfulness into modern medicine and healthcare. He is the creator of the Mindfulness-Based Stress Reduction (MBSR) program. His work has been instrumental in bringing mindfulness and meditation practices into mainstream medicine and psychology.

In sobriety, mindfulness can be a supportive practice, allowing individuals to observe their cravings and emotions without judgment, leading to greater self-regulation and presence. Our upcoming Chapter 17 is exclusively dedicated to living a mindful, sober life, laying out the transformative potential of mindfulness for those seeking a life free from substance use.

Mindfulness brings an engaged awareness to your daily activities, truly experiencing moments with all your senses. Imagine savoring your morning coffee — the aroma, the warmth of the cup in your hands, the taste — as a meditative practice rather than hurriedly gulping it down as you check your phone. This conscious approach to simple tasks rewires your thought processes, helping you cultivate patience, appreciation, and a meaningful connection to the present. Over time, this transformation in how you relate to the external world and your internal landscape can enhance your emotional well-being, offering stability in moments of both joy and adversity.

TIP

To infuse mindfulness into your daily life, start small by choosing one routine activity — like drinking your morning coffee or tea — and commit to experiencing it fully. Focus on the details: the heat radiating through the cup, the intricate dance of flavors on your tongue, and the aroma that lifts your spirits. This trains your brain to apply the same attentive approach to more significant aspects of your life, effectively managing stress and reducing the impulse to turn to substances for comfort or escape. Mindfulness isn't just a practice; it's a way of being that can support your journey to a fulfilling, long-term recovery.

Follow these steps to try the mindful pause:

1. Choose a simple, everyday task like washing your hands, opening a door, or taking a sip of water.

2. Before starting the task, take a deep, slow breath and give full attention to the action you're about to take.

3. As you perform the task, notice all the sensations you can - the temperature, textures, sounds, and any scents.

4. Once the task is complete, take another deep breath and reflect on the experience. What did you notice? Did anything surprise you?

This micro-meditation can be a powerful tool for bringing mindfulness to the mundane, helping you stay grounded and present. It's a practical way to reduce stress and respond to anxiety with a sense of calm.

It's not about perfecting it; it's about practicing awareness and bringing more mindfulness into your day.

For a more in-depth exploration of mindfulness techniques that can support your sober life, be sure to dive into Chapter 15. The skills you nurture there can light up your path to resilience, well-being, and long-term sobriety.

Coping with stress and anxiety

Healthily handling stress and anxiety is a cornerstone of sustaining your sobriety. For instance, meditation offers a sanctuary for your mind, a space to find calm and clarity amidst life's turmoil. Meditating doesn't require a significant time investment — just a few minutes a day can make a substantial difference. It trains you to step back from your thoughts to observe them without judgment, which in turn can help decrease the intensity of stress and anxiety. Additionally, regular physical movement, whether a short daily walk or a yoga session, releases endorphins that naturally improve your mood and combat stress.

However, listening to your inner voice and knowing when these practices are not enough is crucial. Professional mental health support can offer a structured approach to therapy that dives deeper into the root causes of your stress and anxiety. It's not a sign of weakness to seek help — quite the opposite. It demonstrates strength and resilience in acknowledging the need for support. Such professionals can provide personalized strategies beyond general advice, equipping you with the tools to handle life's stressors more effectively.

Part of learning to cope with stress and anxiety involves allowing yourself to feel your emotions fully. It's about not shying away from the discomfort but instead using it as a signal to take action. This might mean taking a mental health day when you're feeling overwhelmed or learning new coping mechanisms like breathing techniques or progressive muscle relaxation. When you give yourself permission to feel and actively seek out coping strategies that resonate with you, it will contribute greatly to the stability of your mental well-being. As you continue on your recovery journey, remember that creating and continuing to refine your personalized wellness routine is a dynamic process that changes with you as you grow.

Your journey to cope with stress and anxiety is deeply personal and unique to your life's rhythm. It's more like gardening than machinery; it requires patience, care, and sometimes, a bit of getting your hands dirty. While meditation and physical activity are fantastic tools for daily maintenance, think of professional support as the expert gardener who can help you unearth the deeper roots, pruning away what no longer serves you. Embracing your emotions as indicators, rather than obstacles, is part of the process — a signal to nurture your well-being with the appropriate practices. This proactive approach can guide you toward a serene mind and a resilient, sober life.

Follow these steps:

1. **Gather your tools:** Find a comfortable spot with your journal or a piece of paper and a pen. If you prefer technology, a digital notepad on your device will work just as well.

2. **Set the scene:** Begin with a quick stretch or a small ritual like sipping a cup of tea to transition into this writing space. This signals to your body and mind that you're entering a reflective time.

3. **Choose power prompts:** Start by writing down a prompt that resonates with you, such as:

   - "Right now, I feel anxious about. . ."

   - "The hardest thoughts for me to let go of are. . ."

   - "When I feel this anxiety, it feels like. . ."

4. **Unleash your thoughts:** Let your thoughts flow onto the page without editing or censoring them. Write everything that comes to mind related to the prompt. This is not about crafting perfect sentences; it's about capturing raw thoughts and feelings.

5. **Dialogue with the page:** Imagine the paper is a trusted friend. What would you tell them about your stress and anxiety? How would they respond? Write down both sides of this conversation.

6. **Create a blueprint for coping:** Reflect on the past strategies that have helped you. Write these down as a reminder, and explore any new ideas that come up, such as:

   - "Taking a brisk walk always clears my head, so I'll schedule one for tomorrow morning."
   - "I remember feeling better after talking to (insert friend's name). I'll reach out to them."

7. **Find actionable insights:** End your journaling session with an actionable insight or commitment to yourself. It could be something like:

   - "I will prioritize my meditation practice because it helps me observe my thoughts."
   - "I will make an appointment with a therapist to explore these feelings further."

8. **Acknowledge the power of writing:** Reflect on how the act of writing has transformed your anxiety into something tangible that you can address and manage. Acknowledge the power of bringing internal struggles into the light and the strength it takes to face them head-on.

Your new journal is designed to engage your mind, provide clarity, and transform the way you cope with stress and anxiety. It's a tangible way to connect with your inner voice and draw out the strategies that best support your path to sobriety and mental well-being.

Seeking professional mental health support and medication

Sometimes, your journey might lead you to seek the expertise of trained mental health professionals such as psychologists, psychiatrists, or other therapists. It's imperative to acknowledge that certain aspects of your mental and emotional well-being can be deeply rooted in past trauma or complex psychological conditions that aren't easily navigated alone. These professionals offer a supportive space to understand and process your emotional reactions to untangle the often-complicated web of past experiences and to provide strategies to cope more effectively with everyday stresses.

In some cases, your path to mental wellness may benefit from the judicious use of medication, which should always be considered in close consultation with a healthcare provider you trust. Medication can be a critical component for some individuals, serving as a stabilizing force while dealing with mood disorders or other underlying mental health issues. It's important to remember that this does not signify dependence or weakness; rather, it is a brave step toward managing your health and improving your quality of life.

Moreover, integrating professional guidance and medication management into your routine should be seen as a proactive measure in maintaining your overall well-being. Whether it's attending regular therapy sessions to navigate life's challenges or finding the right balance of medical treatment, it's about crafting a personalized approach to *your* health that aligns with *your* values and supports *your* goals. Your dedication to seeking help is a testament to your commitment to living a fulfilling, balanced, and healthy life.

TIP

Recognizing when to seek help is a superpower. If you're considering professional mental health support or medication, think of them as tools in a toolkit designed to build a stronger, more resilient version of you. Just like you wouldn't hesitate to wear glasses to see clearly, there's no shame in tapping into professional expertise or medication to gain mental clarity. Set regular check-ins with yourself to assess your mental health; if you notice persistent difficulties, don't wait to reach out for support. Reaching for the tools you need isn't just smart — it's an act of courage and self-care that deserves to be celebrated.

Exploring alternative treatments in recovery

In the evolving landscape of addiction treatment, various alternative therapies have gained attention for their potential role in recovery. These emerging therapies include the use of ketamine, psychedelic medicine, plant medicine, and other innovative treatments. Growing scientific evidence supports the use of alternative therapies and offers guidance on integrating these approaches into your recovery journey.

KETAMINE

Ketamine is a dissociative anesthetic that has been in medical use since the 1970s. Recently, it has shown promise in treating treatment-resistant depression and addiction. Scientific studies indicate that ketamine acts as an NMDA receptor antagonist, which can help alleviate symptoms of depression and reduce cravings in individuals with substance use disorders. A comprehensive review of a decade of research on ketamine psychedelic therapy (KPT) revealed significant improvements in patients struggling with both addiction and depression.

While ketamine itself has potential therapeutic benefits, it's important to note that it can be addictive if misused. The potential for misuse and dependency underscores the necessity for its administration under *strict* medical supervision. When used responsibly within a clinical setting, the risk of addiction is significantly minimized, allowing patients to benefit from its therapeutic effects without the adverse outcomes associated with recreational use.

PSYCHEDELIC MEDICINE

Micordosing psychedelics like LSD, psilocybin (found in magic mushrooms), and MDMA (commonly known as Ecstasy) have been researched extensively for their potential therapeutic effects. These substances are believed to promote neuroplasticity, the brain's ability to reorganize itself by forming new neural connections. This process can be particularly beneficial for individuals dealing with trauma and addiction, as it helps to break maladaptive patterns and foster new, healthier ways of thinking and behaving.

LSD (lysergic acid diethylamide) has been studied for its ability to elicit profound emotional and psychological experiences. These experiences can lead to significant insights and breakthroughs, making it a powerful tool in psychotherapy. Similarly, psilocybin has been shown to reduce symptoms of depression and anxiety, particularly in patients with life-threatening illnesses. Its ability to induce mystical-type experiences has been linked to long-term positive changes in attitudes, mood, and behavior.

MDMA-assisted psychotherapy is another promising area of research. MDMA is known for its empathogenic effects, which enhance feelings of emotional closeness and trust. These effects can create a therapeutic environment where patients feel safe to explore and process traumatic experiences. Clinical trials have demonstrated that MDMA-assisted therapy can lead to substantial and sustained reductions in PTSD (post-traumatic stress syndrome) symptoms, which is often a co-occurring condition with substance use disorders.

Modern double-blind, randomized controlled trials have provided rich evidence supporting the efficacy of these compounds. A recent study found that psilocybin treatment led to significant reductions in alcohol dependence, with effects lasting up to nine months. Research on MDMA-assisted psychotherapy has shown impressive results, with many participants experiencing significant improvements in their mental health that persist long after the treatment sessions have ended.

The growing body of evidence underscores the potential of psychedelics to transform traditional approaches to addiction and mental health treatment. By promoting neuroplasticity and enabling emotional breakthroughs, these substances offer a unique pathway to healing and personal growth. It's important to consider as with any treatment, it's *crucial* to approach psychedelic therapy under the guidance of trained professionals to ensure safety and efficacy.

PLANT MEDICINE

Plant-based treatments such as Ayahuasca and Ibogaine have traditional roots in various cultures and have been explored for their potential to treat addiction. Ayahuasca, a brew made from Amazonian plants, is known for its intense psychoactive properties and has been used in ceremonial contexts to promote healing and self-discovery. Research indicates that Ayahuasca can significantly reduce alcohol consumption rates among users. For example, a cross-sectional study comparing Ayahuasca users to a normative sample found significantly lower last-year and last-month alcohol consumption among the users.

Similarly, ibogaine, derived from the iboga plant, has shown promise in interrupting addiction cycles, particularly for opioids, by modulating brain neurotransmitters and reducing withdrawal symptoms. A study on participants undergoing opioid detoxification with ibogaine reported marked reductions in withdrawal and craving scores. Despite concerns related to its cardiotoxicity, the evidence supporting ibogaine's potential for treating substance dependence is growing. Its ability to transition opioid and cocaine abusers from dependence to abstinence points to its role as a powerful therapeutic agent.

Broader literature suggests that the community and ceremonial aspects of these plant-based treatments also play a significant role in their efficacy. The settings in which these substances are typically administered — often involving structured support and guided introspection — can enhance the therapeutic outcomes. This underscores the importance of a holistic approach to addiction treatment, one that integrates medical, psychological, and community support mechanisms.

As alternative treatments gain more scientific validation, they offer new avenues for individuals seeking to overcome addiction. Approaching these therapies under professional supervision is crucial to ensure safety and maximize their potential benefits. Integrating plant-based treatments into a comprehensive recovery plan can provide a transformative path toward healing, underscoring the need for continued research and clinical application.

ALTERNATIVE TREATMENTS

Other non-classic psychedelics, like MDMA, are also being studied for their ability to support addiction recovery. MDMA-assisted psychotherapy, for example, has shown potential in alleviating severe PTSD, which is often a co-occurring condition with substance use disorders.

Scientific evidence

If you are interested in these alternative treatments, research is paramount. Studies have demonstrated that these substances can significantly impact brain function, emotional regulation, and overall mental health. For instance, the following treatments have been shown to be effective:

>> **Ketamine:** Studies have shown its efficacy in treatment-resistant depression and addiction.

>> **Psilocybin:** Research has highlighted its potential to reduce anxiety and depression in terminally ill patients, which can translate to broader applications in mental health and addiction treatment.

>> **MDMA:** Clinical trials have demonstrated its effectiveness in treating PTSD, which can indirectly support recovery from addiction.

The importance of open-mindedness in recovery

If you explore these alternative treatments, it's crucial to stay open-minded and focused on your recovery needs. Alternative treatments and medication are controversial in some twelve-step circles, even though the founder of AA, Bill Wilson, had his own psychedelic experience that led to the creation of AA. It's important to consider all options and choose what resonates with you, always in consultation with your healthcare provider.

In previous sections, we discussed the importance of seeking help and support with trauma work (as highlighted in Chapter 3). Addressing underlying trauma can be a pivotal element of your recovery journey, and integrating alternative treatments under professional guidance can provide additional support in this process.

As you navigate your path to long-term recovery, remember that your journey is unique to you. You can build a recovery plan supporting your long-term well-being and personal growth by staying open to new possibilities and focusing on your needs.

Finding support

If you need professional mental health support or medication, there are several avenues you can explore to find the right help for you:

>> **Primary care provider:** Your first step could be to speak with your primary care physician. They can provide initial

guidance, diagnose potential issues, refer you to specialists, and help manage medications if needed.

>> **Mental health professionals:** For more specialized care, consider consulting psychologists, health counselors, or psychiatrists. As of 2023, six states — Louisiana, New Mexico, Illinois, Iowa, Idaho, and Colorado — have enacted laws that allow specially trained licensed psychologists to prescribe certain types of medication. Therapists can provide therapy, while psychiatrists are medical doctors who can prescribe and manage medication and provide therapy.

>> **Insurance company:** If you have health insurance, check your provider's website or call their customer service for a list of covered mental health services and providers in your network.

>> **Online directories:** Utilize online directories and mental health organizations to find therapists, counselors, and other mental health professionals. Platforms like Psychology Today and GoodTherapy allow you to search by location, specialty, and insurance.

>> **Employee Assistance Programs (EAP):** If you're employed, your workplace might offer an EAP, which can provide confidential assessments, short-term counseling, referrals, and follow-up services.

>> **Local clinics and hospitals:** Community clinics and hospitals often have mental health departments with various services. They may offer sliding-scale fees based on your income.

>> **Telehealth services:** Telehealth services provide therapy and medical consultations online if you prefer or require remote options.

>> **Support groups:** Look for support groups where you can connect with others facing similar challenges. Sometimes, these groups are led by a mental health professional.

>> **National helplines:** If you're in crisis or need immediate help, contact national helplines like the National Suicide Prevention Lifeline (1-800-273-TALK) for support and guidance.

>> **Educational resources:** Educate yourself about mental health through reputable sources such as the National Alliance on Mental Illness (NAMI) or the Substance Abuse and Mental Health Services Administration (SAMHSA).

REMEMBER

Seeking help is a sign of strength, not weakness. It's important to take action early to address your mental health needs effectively.

Holistic Approaches to Physical Health

Staying on the path of sobriety is not just about breaking free from the grips of substance dependency; it's about rejuvenating and strengthening your physical health through a holistic lens. Understanding the intricate relationship between your body and overall well-being is pivotal to healing and supporting your recovery. It's about cultivating habits that nourish your body, mind, and spirit, creating a synergy that fosters a balanced and healthy life.

Focusing on holistic approaches encourages you to look at your health from a broader perspective. This involves considering how your diet, exercise regimen, and sleep patterns can profoundly impact your sobriety journey. Food, for instance, should be considered *fuel* and *medicine*, with mindful eating practices that help you recognize the effects of various foods on your body and emotions. Similarly, physical activity becomes more than just a way to stay fit; it's a vital tool for managing stress, improving mood, and boosting mental clarity. Regular exercise, whether a quick ten-minute workout or an extended session fitting into your busy schedule, is instrumental in building resilience and physical strength to face the challenges of everyday life.

In terms of understanding your body's needs, recognizing the importance of lab work and genetic propensities can be eye-opening, as read in chapter 6. Such insights can guide you to adopt functional medicine approaches tailored to your unique physiological makeup. This approach goes beyond traditional medicine by addressing the root causes of health issues rather than merely treating symptoms. Embracing these practices leads to a more informed, personalized wellness routine that can evolve with you as you progress in your sobriety. Reflecting on these elements of health and incorporating practices like mindfulness, meditation, and appropriate medical support builds a solid foundation from which you can grow and maintain a life of sobriety enriched by physical vitality and emotional balance.

REMEMBER

In your sobriety journey, taking a holistic view of your physical health is crucial. By focusing on a balanced diet, consistent exercise, and restorative sleep, you address the needs of your body, mind, and spirit. Don't overlook the power of lab work and genetic insights to personalize your approach to wellness, aiming not just to treat symptoms but to find and address the underlying causes. This comprehensive care is the cornerstone of building long-term, healthy recovery.

Your physical health: the role of lab tests

Understanding the details of your body's functioning can be incredibly empowering in long-term recovery. Lab tests can unlock a wealth of information about your nutritional status, hormonal balance, and genetic predispositions. Here's how you can use this data to tailor your wellness practices:

>> **Nutrient levels:** Monitoring your nutrient levels is key for supporting recovery, with vitamin D being essential for mood and immune health; B vitamins for energy and brain function; magnesium for stress reduction and metabolic health; and iron for preventing fatigue and improving concentration. Adequate levels of these nutrients can significantly enhance physical and mental well-being during your journey to sobriety.

>> **Hormone panels:** Hormonal imbalances can affect everything from metabolism to mood. Tests that measure thyroid

function, cortisol levels, and sex hormones can provide insights for addressing potential imbalances holistically. Hormone panels are crucial in managing recovery from addiction because hormones regulate critical functions that can be disrupted by substance use. Evaluating cortisol helps us understand your stress response, which is often heightened in addiction. Thyroid hormones shape your metabolism and energy levels, influencing mood and overall vitality. Sex hormones affect not only reproductive health but also mood and motivation.

>> **Metabolic markers:** Assessing your metabolic markers like blood sugar, cholesterol, and liver function is crucial in addiction recovery. Substance use can disrupt these levels, affecting overall health. Regular testing ensures that your recovery plan addresses these imbalances, promoting a healthier lifestyle free from alcohol.

>> **Food sensitivity and allergy tests:** Identifying food sensitivities and allergies is particularly important. Substance use can alter your body's response to certain foods, potentially causing inflammation and discomfort that you might have previously masked with alcohol or substances. By pinpointing which foods don't agree with you, you can tailor your diet to avoid these triggers. This proactive step aids in managing energy levels and reducing inflammation, which is essential for healing and maintaining a body free from the effects of substances.

>> **Genetic testing:** Some services offer genetic testing that can highlight potential health risks and how your body may respond to certain medications, nutrients, and activities. You would also be able to see how your dopamine receptors and AKT1, ALDH2, and OPRM1 genes work.

>> **Gut health assessments:** Evaluating your gut health through assessments such as stool analyses is key to addiction recovery. Substance use can disrupt the delicate balance of your gut microbiome, negatively impacting digestion, immune function, and even mental health — all of which are critical areas in the journey toward sobriety. Understanding and nurturing gut health can support your body's recovery and contribute positively to your overall well-being.

>> **Toxicity screenings:** Screenings for heavy metals and other toxins can be beneficial if you've had past exposure to substances. Detoxifying your body can be a significant step in holistic healing.

When considering lab tests, it's wise to consult with healthcare professionals who can provide guidance based on your specific health history and recovery journey. This could be your primary care physician or an online functional medicine practitioner who is trained to interpret these tests within the context of your overall health and lifestyle.

By integrating lab tests into your holistic health approach, you can craft a wellness routine that's truly tailored to you. This isn't about chasing an ideal of perfection but about finding what works for your body and supports your recovery. Learning and understanding your body is a process of discovery, one in which you learn to listen and respond to your body's signals with care and precision.

TIP

Discussing your lab work with your primary doctor is important and helps you be both informed and strategic. Here's a concise yet thorough approach:

>> **Research:** Before your appointment, gather evidence-based studies related to the lab tests you're interested in. For instance, studies linking addiction recovery to changes in hormone levels or gut health can be compelling.

>> **Documentation:** Bring a copy of the study to share with your doctor. Highlight or note down the parts that directly relate to your situation.

>> **History and concerns:** Be ready to discuss your history with substance use disorder and express your concerns about how it may have impacted your health, including your mental health as well. Mentioning specific symptoms or health challenges will help articulate the need for testing.

>> **Specific tests:** Clearly state which tests you are interested in. For example: "I'm interested in having my estrogen, progesterone, and testosterone levels checked due to their role in mood regulation and overall health, which I understand can be affected by long-term substance use."

>> **Benefits:** Explain how obtaining these lab results can contribute to fine-tuning your recovery plan and preventing relapse by monitoring critical health indicators.

>> **Open dialogue:** Encourage an open dialog by saying something like, "I read this study about the significant role of the microbiome in addiction recovery, and it made me consider that we might be overlooking some factors that could help with my health challenges."

>> **Plan B:** Be prepared for the possibility that your primary doctor may not order the tests. If this happens, you can discuss alternative options, such as seeing a specialist or using online lab services that allow you to order tests independently, often at a reasonable fee.

Approach the conversation with respect for your doctor's expertise while also advocating for your health needs. Your goal is to partner with your healthcare provider to ensure you're on the most effective path to your personal sustained recovery.

Prioritizing regular exercise in sobriety

Understanding the role of regular exercise in achieving long-term sobriety is critical. Exercise is an anchor for your well-being, providing a cascade of benefits extending well beyond the apparent physical health improvements. Each step you take, each weight you lift, is a step away from previous habits and a stride toward a healthier you. Beyond the obvious physical health improvements, exercise provides a range of benefits that support the recovery process. Scientific research has shown that regular physical activity can elevate mood, reduce stress, and improve sleep — all key factors in maintaining sobriety. Exercise is known to stimulate the release of endorphins, chemicals in the brain that act as natural painkillers and mood elevators, which can help combat the feelings of depression that sometimes accompany substance use disorder recovery.

Regular exercise also contributes to better stress management. Physical exertion acts as a natural outlet for stress and, over time, can improve the body's resilience to stressors, which is essential for reducing the risk of relapse. Additionally, regular physical activity has been linked to improved sleep patterns. Better sleep not only aids in physical recovery but also helps regulate emotions and improve cognitive function, which is critical for those in recovery.

The type of exercise is less critical than the consistency of your practice. Short, frequent sessions can be just as effective as longer workouts, which is encouraging for those with busy schedules. Consistent physical activity can help redirect the focus from cravings or triggers to positive and proactive self-care.

Recognizing the mental and emotional gains from regular exercise is also important. As you progress in your fitness journey, you develop muscle and mental fortitude, learning to overcome challenges and setting the stage for similar victories in your sobriety journey.

Exercise in sobriety isn't just about self-improvement; it's a pathway to self-discovery. As you push yourself to new limits, you'll uncover inner strength you may not have known existed. This journey into physical activity becomes a metaphor for your journey in sobriety — overcoming obstacles, enduring pain, and celebrating victories, no matter how small they seem. It's about establishing a routine that reinforces your sobriety and builds upon the foundation of recovery. Each drop of sweat is a testament to your dedication, and each completed exercise session is a victory in your ongoing commitment to a sober life.

Embrace exercise as a trusted companion in your sober life. Appreciate the days when motivation flows, and the workouts seem effortless and draw strength from the days when you'd rather do anything else than exercise, yet do it anyway. Each choice to prioritize exercise is a choice to prioritize your sobriety, health, and, ultimately, your life. Regular exercise is a fundamental component of a holistic recovery strategy, playing a pivotal role in preserving and enhancing the quality of your sobriety.

REMEMBER

Regular exercise is essential for long-term sobriety. It's a powerful tool that enhances both physical and mental health, aiding in stress reduction, mood improvement, and better sleep. Consistency in your physical activity is key, not the type or length of exercise. Embrace the mental resilience and self-discovery that comes with pushing your physical limits. Prioritize exercise to reinforce your commitment to sobriety and build a strong foundation for recovery.

JOURNEY WITH MOVEMENT WITH KATE

First, I dropped the word exercise from my vernacular and replaced it with the word movement. I remind myself I am not trying to win an Olympic medal. I don't need to train and "work out." I need to move my body. Movement is literally medicine. I put a treadmill in my bedroom to make my new habit obvious and accessible. Each day, when I come home from work, I tell myself I will get on it and walk. On the days I work from home, I wear athletic sneakers around the house to prompt more purposeful movement in my day-to-day habits. Wearing sneakers in my house also makes jumping on the treadmill an easy transition. (I eliminate any barriers I can think of because I like to make excuses to sit on my butt.)

Moving my body solves multiple problems at once. I can kickstart the endorphins in my brain and improve my mood while boosting my confidence, knowing that I am doing something good for myself. I experience less back and shoulder pain and sleep better. I also learned to use this time to meditate in motion. I started listening to podcasts and audiobooks while I walked and really contemplated the information I was hearing. Some days, I listen to soothing music when I have a lot of thoughts to process. Movement really helps me with anxiety and impulsiveness. When I feel the urge to numb out with booze or food or shopping, I know I need to get moving.

Believe it or not, I now view my treadmill as a tool that really helps my recovery. It is no longer a torture device that prompts feelings of dread. I don't equate the treadmill to bikini season; I see it now as a place to go when I want to drop into my body and process emotions. Sound corny? It is because I am no longer in the business of browbeating myself into better habits. I am gently and purposefully moving toward a new way of being. I'd rather be a little corny than a lot drunk.

(continued)

(continued)

Today, when I coach clients on sobriety, I encourage practical movement methods to start. Take the stairs. Park farther away and walk. Get outside and make a lap around your neighborhood. Movement begets more movement. You will increase your intensity and frequency as time passes because it feels good, not because you feel obligated. Dance around your apartment to Britney Spears. Do wall push-ups. Stretch. Do some squats during mundane chores. Keep your athletic shoes on and create opportunities to move.

One final thought on movement is that it allows me to witness my body's abilities and have gratitude for them. Look how my legs can carry me, and my spine holds me upright. Notice how I can swing my arms and move my neck. It's important for me to have gratitude for a body that I poisoned for years with alcohol and witness its resiliency and strength in recovery. The human body is a miracle; daily movement reminds me of this.

Nutritional practices for recovery

What you fuel your body with is just as important as your physical activities. Nutrition in recovery isn't just about following a diet — it's about understanding how different foods affect your mood, energy levels, and cravings. Journaling your food intake and its impacts empowers you to make informed choices and can help you identify triggers or deficiencies hindering your progress. You pave the way for a clearer mind and a more resilient body through mindful eating habits and a balanced diet.

Your journey to recovery is unique, and so are your nutritional needs. You may find that certain foods that are generally considered healthy might not sit well with you, causing discomfort or even cravings for substances you're working to avoid. By tracking your meals and emotional state, you'll notice patterns that reveal which foods support your sobriety and which ones to limit. This personalized approach to nutrition allows you to take charge of your recovery, one meal at a time.

Incorporating various nutrient-dense foods into your diet is crucial in healing your body and mind. Seeking professional guidance can be immensely beneficial. A dietitian knowledgeable in recovery can help tailor a food plan supporting your situation. They can introduce you to delicious meals and provide the vitamins and minerals essential for your recovery. Plus, they can offer strategies for meal prepping, managing cravings, and making nutritious choices when dining out or on the go.

TIP

Keep a detailed food diary — not just a list of what you eat, but also notes on how you feel physically and emotionally afterward. This can help you connect the dots between your diet and your recovery experience. Discover which foods fuel your body and elevate your mood and which ones might lead to unwanted cravings or energy crashes. Treat this diary as a compass that guides you to a diet tailored to support your unique recovery process. By becoming an expert on your body's responses to different foods, you're actively shaping your road to a healthier you.

Reduce cravings

It is critical to ingest amino acids, which play a crucial role in the long-term recovery from substance use disorders. They're often referred to as the building blocks of protein, which, in turn, is the building block of life. Amino acids are fundamental for the production of neurotransmitters, which were discussed earlier in the chapter. Neurotransmitters are the brain's chemical messengers that significantly affect mood regulation and cravings.

If you want to achieve stable moods throughout the day and reduce your cravings is paramount, then amino acids are your new best friends. These neurotransmitters, including serotonin, dopamine, and norepinephrine, are affected by substance use. Amino acids from dietary protein can help restore balance in these neurotransmitters. Eating foods rich in amino acids every three or four hours helps maintain a steady stream of these building blocks, stabilizing blood sugar levels and mood and reducing the urge for substances by providing the brain with the resources it needs to heal and function optimally.

Nutrient-dense foods high in amino acids include:

>> **Chicken breast:** Chicken breasts are a lean protein source high in the amino acid tryptophan, which the body converts into serotonin.

>> **Salmon:** Salmon is rich in omega-3 fatty acids and provides a full range of amino acids, aiding in brain function and recovery.

>> **Eggs:** All nine essential amino acids are particularly rich in leucine, which is crucial for muscle repair and growth.

>> **Quinoa:** Quinoa is a complete protein, meaning it contains *all* essential amino acids; it's also high in fiber and nutrients.

>> **Greek yogurt:** Packed with amino acids, Greek yogurt also has the added benefit of probiotics for gut health, which can influence mental well-being.

Creating and maintaining a protein journal can be a key component of recovery to avoid relapse. It serves as a daily log to ensure regular intake of amino acid–rich foods and to monitor how changes in diet correlate with mood and craving levels. This practice also encourages your mindfulness practice about nutrition and its impact on your sobriety. Tracking protein intake ensures that you're supporting your brain chemistry actively and may help identify patterns between what you eat and how you feel, allowing for more informed dietary choices that support recovery.

REMEMBER

Recovery is a path filled with learning and growth. As you embrace these nutritional practices, be kind to yourself and recognize that it's a process of trial and error. Celebrate the small victories, like reaching for a fruit instead of a candy bar or cooking a wholesome meal at home. These seemingly simple actions accumulate to create profound changes in your overall health and well-being, setting a solid foundation for a life in recovery.

Other treatments to support your recovery

Your journey through recovery is deeply personal, and when it comes to the role of medication and treatments, it's important to approach it with care and professionalism. Standing by the principle that medication should be taken when necessary and under a doctor's supervision is a responsible stance ensuring safety and effectiveness.

Gaining access to mental health support within the context of addiction and recovery is vital. Proper medical attention cannot be overstated. Medications that are closely monitored and taken as directed can provide necessary support. This is not just a safety measure but also a way to honor the complex needs of every individual's recovery process.

Exploring GLP-1 for addiction

In recent years, the scientific community has turned its attention to glucagon-like peptide-1 (GLP-1) receptor agonists as a potential treatment for addiction. Originally developed to manage diabetes and obesity, GLP-1 receptor agonists have shown promise in regulating brain functions related to reward and addiction.

GLP-1 is a hormone that plays a key role in glucose metabolism and appetite control. Researchers have discovered that GLP-1 receptors are not only found in the gut but also in the brain, particularly in regions involved in addiction and reward pathways, such as the nucleus accumbens and the ventral tegmental area.

Studies have shown that GLP-1 receptor activation can reduce alcohol consumption and mitigate drug-seeking behaviors in animal models. These findings suggest that GLP-1 receptor agonists could potentially modulate the brain's reward system, making them a promising candidate for treating addiction. However, it is important to note that research on GLP-1 receptor agonists in addiction treatment is still in its early stages. Most of the evidence comes from animal studies, and more human trials are needed to establish the efficacy and safety of GLP-1 receptor agonists for addiction.

Other healing paths

Exploring other healing paths, such as MDMA-assisted therapy and psychedelic medicine, is indeed a growing area of interest in the field of addiction and recovery. (MDMA [3,4-methylenedioxy methamphetamine] is also known as Ecstasy.) For example, MDMA-assisted therapy has been researched for its potential to treat PTSD (post-traumatic stress disorder), which can be co-occurring with substance use disorders. The idea is that MDMA, in a controlled therapeutic setting, may enhance the effectiveness of psychotherapy by reducing fear and increasing trust, potentially leading to breakthroughs in emotional processing.

These treatments are being explored in clinical trials and are not widely available as standard care. Their legality varies by region and they are usually administered under strict clinical supervision, with a focus on set and setting — meaning the individual's mental state and the environment in which the treatment takes place.

It's crucial to highlight that while there is growing evidence for these treatments, they are not a one-size-fits-all solution and come with their own set of risks and considerations. Therefore, they should only be considered when legal, ethical, and safety standards are fully observed. In any case, you should be encouraged to seek out and adhere to evidence-based treatments licensed healthcare professionals provide. Open dialogue with healthcare providers about all forms of treatment, including cutting-edge therapies like MDMA-assisted therapy, psychedelic medicine, and GLP-1 receptor agonists, is essential to navigating recovery with informed consent and support.

REMEMBER

If you're considering alternative therapies such as GLP-1 receptor agonists, MDMA-assisted therapy, or psychedelic medicine to support your recovery, it's essential to prioritize safety and legality. Always consult with a healthcare professional and ensure any treatment is part of a structured and supervised program. Stay informed about the latest clinical trials and research to understand the potential benefits and risks. These therapies may offer new hope, but they also require a commitment to follow guidelines and to only engage in such treatments under professional care within a legal framework. Recovery is a multi-faceted journey, and exploring new treatments should always be done with mindfulness and ethical consideration.

The role of sleep in physical well-being

Sleep is a crucial element of any wellness routine, often being the unsung hero of physical and mental recovery, especially on the path of long-term sobriety. Your body utilizes sleep to perform vital functions that repair and rejuvenate tissues, clear toxins from your brain, and strengthen your immune system. By ensuring you get the recommended seven to nine hours of quality sleep each night, you're allowing your body to reset, which can be particularly beneficial after the stress of addiction and the recovery process.

When you're well-rested, your decision-making skills improve, and your willpower is strengthened — both essential for maintaining sobriety. Sleep deprivation, on the other hand, can lead to increased cravings and a heightened stress response, both of which can be triggering for those in recovery. By prioritizing sleep, you're effectively equipping yourself with an extra layer of defense against relapse. Think of sleep as an investment in your future, quieting the noise of the day and preparing you to face tomorrow's challenges with resilience and clarity.

Quality sleep influences your emotional stability. A rested brain is more capable of managing moods and regulating emotions, which can be tumultuous during sobriety. This emotional steadiness helps in mitigating the anxiety and depression symptoms that are often associated with withdrawal and early recovery phases. Achieving a restorative night's sleep isn't just about quantity; it entails cultivating a serene sleeping environment and adhering to routines that promote relaxation and calmness before bedtime. Embrace practices like dimming the lights, reducing screen time, and perhaps incorporating meditation or gentle stretching to signal to your body that it's time to wind down.

Finally, sleep plays a pivotal role in physical performance and recovery. Whether you're engaging in light exercise as a beginner or following a more intense regimen, sleep supports muscle repair and growth. You'll notice that your energy levels are higher on days following a good night's sleep, and your workouts may feel more effective. During sleep, your body does much of the work to rebuild from the physical exertions of the day, making it an indispensable part of your wellness toolkit in sobriety. Simply put, to thrive physically in your recovery journey, sleep cannot be an afterthought; it must be a priority, on par with your nutritional and exercise habits.

TIP

Commit to treating your bedtime with the same importance as a key meeting or a doctor's appointment. Establish a sleep sanctuary free of electronics, use soothing colors and comfortable bedding, and set a consistent sleep schedule. Consider incorporating a wind-down ritual, like reading or listening to calm music, to cue your body that it's time for rest. By honoring your need for restful sleep, you're building a foundation of resilience that supports every step you take on the path to long-term sobriety. Remember, sleep isn't just a pause from your daily life; it's a vital act of self-preservation that replenishes your strength and fortifies your resolve.

NOW SLEEPING SOBER WITH KATARINA

My journey to better sleep didn't happen overnight. It took me nearly three years into my recovery to realize how essential a role rest played in my well-being. My sleep used to be scattered and unrefreshing, especially during the years I was drinking and even after I stopped. I'd toss and turn, my mind racing with a never-ending to-do list and regrets from the past.

I knew something had to change when my recovery began to feel like a constant uphill battle. I was always tired and irritable, and my cravings were harder to manage. That's when I started to connect the dots between my sleep habits and my sobriety.

First on my list was the blue light from screens. Research has shown that it can mess with your sleep by tricking your brain into thinking it's still daytime. I decided to wear blue-light-blocking glasses in the evenings, which helped me wind down before bed.

Next, I tackled the invisible culprit — electromagnetic fields, or EMFs. I'd read about how the signals from cell phones and Wi-Fi could disrupt sleep, so I began turning off my devices and even the whole house's Internet an hour before bedtime. Surprisingly, I noticed a change within a few days; my sleep was deeper, and I woke up feeling more rested.

But it wasn't just about cutting out the bad but also about adding in the good. Establishing a bedtime routine became my new priority. I swapped late-night shows for a soothing herbal tea and aimed to be in bed by 10 PM, a full two hours earlier than my old midnight habit. Consistency has been key. Even during recovery meetings in the evening, I stick to my routine and catch that crucial sleep window.

Now, six years into my sobriety journey, living with my boyfriend, who respects my sleep schedule, I can't imagine going back to my old ways. He may stay up later, but my rest is non-negotiable. It's as important to my recovery as my support meetings — both are non-negotiable.

My sleep transformation was not merely about changing one habit; it was about honoring my body's need for rest as a pillar of my recovery. It's a sacred time, a daily ritual that says, "I care about my well-being." And with that, I wake up to my sobriety each morning, renewed and ready to face the day.

REMEMBER

Sleep isn't just a nightly hiatus; it's a restorative necessity for both mind and body, especially in recovery. Establishing a sleep routine free from blue light and EMF disruptions is critical. Embrace the stillness of the night, use it to recharge fully, and you'll wake up with renewed vigor to face each day's journey with clarity. Your sleep is your secret weapon in maintaining your sobriety and living your best life in recovery.

Discovering Emotional Wellness

Emotional wellness represents a deeply personal journey of balance and understanding. In sobriety, recognizing and accepting your emotions is essential. It's about adeptly navigating life's varied emotional landscapes, armed with resilience and grace. Emotional wellness goes beyond feeling good; it's the skillful regulation of emotions, allowing for effective stress management, recovery from setbacks, and savoring your successes. By learning the art of emotional regulation, you can better cope with stress, recover from disappointments, and enjoy the highs of your achievements.

Developing a wellness routine tailored to your unique needs is vital. This routine can incorporate practices like mindfulness, ensuring restful sleep, engaging in regular physical activity, and pursuing activities that allow for creative expression, like journaling or art. Such a routine aims to create an environment where emotional wellness can thrive, supporting a more harmonious relationship with your thoughts and emotions.

Each stride in your recovery, no matter how small, deserves recognition. By valuing your growth and the effort you've invested in your recovery, you reinforce positive behaviors and fortify your commitment to a sober life.

Emotional wellness exercise: Identifying and defining your emotions

This exercise is designed to help you become more aware of your emotions and understand them better. Emotional wellness is about recognizing, accepting, and healthily managing your feelings. By becoming more attuned to your emotions, you'll be better prepared to deal with the ups and downs of life, especially as you continue on your sobriety path.

Follow these steps:

1. **List your emotions:** Start by listing different emotions you experience throughout the week. Don't judge or try to change these feelings; simply note them down. Examples may include:

   - Happiness

   - Sadness

- Anger
- Fear
- Disappointment
- Excitement
- Frustration
- Loneliness

2. **Define each emotion:** Next to each emotion you've listed, write a brief definition or describe a situation that typically triggers this emotion for you. For example:

   - **Happiness:** A sense of joy and contentment, like spending time with loved ones.

   - **Sadness:** A feeling of sorrow is often triggered by loss or disappointment.

   - **Anger:** A strong feeling of annoyance, displeasure, or hostility might arise from feeling mistreated or frustrated by a situation.

3. **Reflect on the emotions:** Reflect on each emotion and how it affects you. Ask yourself:

   - How does this emotion feel physically in my body?
   - What thoughts tend to accompany this emotion?
   - How do I typically respond or behave when I feel this emotion?
   - What healthy coping strategies can I use to manage this emotion?

4. **Develop coping strategies:** Finally, for each emotion, write down a coping strategy or an activity you can do to manage that emotion positively. These might include:

   - **Happiness:** I share my joy with others or note what caused it to be repeated in the future.

   - **Sadness:** Allow myself to feel and express sadness, perhaps by journaling or talking to a friend.

   - **Anger:** Use deep breathing techniques or take a walk to cool down.

Remember, the goal of this exercise isn't to eliminate your emotions but to understand and manage them better. Emotional wellness is a critical component of recovery, and by practicing awareness and regulation of your feelings, you'll reinforce your sobriety with every step.

This exercise is just a starting point. As you get more comfortable identifying and dealing with your emotions, you can expand your list and your strategies. Each emotion is a signal, and by listening to what they tell you, you can navigate life's challenges with greater ease and resilience.

Understanding emotional regulation

Emotional regulation is the cornerstone of your emotional wellness. It *requires* you to be candid with your feelings and allows space to acknowledge and express them. In the sober journey, you might find that feelings you once numbed with substances now come to the fore. Engage with these emotions mindfully, using meditation, journaling, and deep breathing exercises to navigate through them. Remember, it's not just about controlling your emotions but honoring and learning from them. By processing these emotions, you can reclaim the power over your reactions and responses to the world around you.

Embracing your emotions is essential for fostering resilience and maintaining your sobriety. As you embark on this path, allow yourself the grace to feel without judgment. You may experience a spectrum of emotions, from joy to sorrow, and that's perfectly normal. Your task is to witness these emotions without letting them define or overwhelm you. Emotional regulation provides a framework to understand these complex feelings and adapt to them constructively. With practice, you'll become adept at recognizing what triggers certain emotions and develop strategies to maintain equilibrium even in the face of life's ups and downs.

The role of sleep and physiological well-being cannot be understated when it comes to emotional regulation. Prioritize rest as it is pivotal in processing and reacting to emotions. Lack of sleep can amplify negativity and reduce your capacity for emotional management. Supplementing your resting routines with physical activity is equally important, as exercise profoundly stabilizes mood. Embrace routines that include soothing and energizing activities, like yoga or brisk walking, to promote balance and enhance your emotional regulation capabilities.

Your journey to mastering emotional regulation is a deeply personal one. While common strategies can be a great starting point, crafting a routine that resonates with your unique needs is critical. Emotional mindfulness, a term that signifies an increased awareness of both the presence and the role of emotions, can lead to more deliberate responses to situations that once might have prompted an automatic reaction. Self-expression through art, music, or dance can also be a potent tool for managing emotions. By actively engaging in emotional regulation, you are equipping yourself with the skills to lead a more centered, sober life filled with understanding and self-compassion.

TIP

Create a brief "emotion response plan" to navigate your intense feelings:

>> **Identify triggers:** Note what ignites your emotions for a week.

>> **Define coping mechanisms:** Link each emotion to a healthy coping action, like meditation for stress or a walk for sadness.

>> **Set a consistent sleep routine:** Establish and maintain a regular sleep schedule.

>> **Incorporate physical activity:** Daily exercise, such as walking, should be non-negotiable for mood balance.

>> **Engage in daily mindfulness:** Spend time each day observing your emotions without judgment to cultivate awareness.

>> **Adjust as needed:** Monitor the effectiveness of your strategies and make changes where necessary.

These steps are a part of your emotional toolkit, empowering you to honor and manage your emotions for a more balanced, sober life.

Creating your personalized wellness routine

Your personalized wellness routine is about tuning inward, listening to your body and mind and recognizing what practices contribute to your sense of well-being. Start by considering areas in your life that could use more attention or improvement. You may want to focus on improving your sleep quality, managing stress more effectively, or increasing your physical activity. Reflect on what brings you joy and peace, whether it's a hobby, spending time with loved ones, or simply taking a moment to breathe and be still. We will go further into this topic in Chapter 11.

Evaluating your current habits is a lifelong journey in sober life. Your next step is to examine your diet and ask yourself if it nourishes your body. Does it? How do you feel when you eat? Are you aware of what you place into your body? Consider implementing nutritional practices that support recovery, like journaling your foods and noting how they affect you physically and emotionally. Physical activity can also boost your mental health, so explore different types of exercises to see what fits into your lifestyle — anything from yoga to a quick ten-minute home workout can do wonders.

Mindfulness should be a cornerstone of your wellness routine as it can help you maintain emotional regulation. Experiment with various forms of mindfulness exercises — perhaps start with a five-minute meditation session each morning or practice mindful eating during your meals. Listen to your body and your emotions; they will guide you toward the activities that serve you best. Remember, this routine is about self-care, so be flexible and kind to yourself as you find what works for you.

Lastly, your wellness routine isn't set in stone. It needs to evolve as you do. Be open to trying new things and adjust as necessary. Maybe a new type of workout will inspire you, or adding a gratitude journal will offer a fresh perspective. Whatever you choose, the goal is to develop a routine that supports every aspect of your well-being, strengthens your sobriety, and ultimately becomes a source of comfort and strength in your daily life.

TRANSFORMS WITH A PERSONAL ROUTINE WITH JOSH

I moved back home to San Diego, where the ocean kisses the shores, and my folks — well, they're getting used to the idea. It's been a year since I kicked the bottle, swapping bar nights for morning jogs, caffeine for more sleep, and takeout for home-cooked proteins. I'm Josh, fresh out of college with an engineering degree in one hand and a non-alcoholic beer in the other.

My parents didn't throw a welcome party when I showed up with bags full of laundry and a heart full of hope. They knew, though, that it was the best shot for their son to keep climbing on that sobriety ladder.

Let me tell you, the job market's a beast. Tech companies want fresh meat but seasoned experience — go figure. That's why my wellness is my priority. Without that crutch, I can't afford to lose myself again after this year of discovering who I am.

I started with the small stuff — ditching my daily coffee at 6 AM and eating right. I stash protein bars everywhere — in my car, my old room that now feels new, and even in the pockets of my running shorts. It's like being a squirrel gearing up for winter — except winter's an urge that could pop up when I least expect it, and those bars are my shield.

Then there's tennis — my new best friend. It's the only time I chase after something that doesn't leave me with regret. The guys from my sober home group have become my cheering squad, my brothers. We hit the gym like it's our job, maybe because, in a way, it is.

This routine of mine is not just about staying busy. It's about tuning into what my body and mind tell me. It's about making sure I'm more than okay. I'm thriving, day by day, step by step. And it's not set in stone — it changes as I change. It reflects the life I'm building, sober and strong.

TIP

Create a wellness routine to support sobriety. Start small. Replace a habit that doesn't serve you with one that does. If you're like Josh, swap out your morning coffee for extra sleep to kickstart your day with clearer focus. Keep healthy snacks like protein bars handy to combat cravings and maintain energy. Dive into a new physical activity that excites you, like tennis, and find your community, whether it's at the gym or a sober group. This isn't just about filling time; it's about actively shaping a life that echoes your dedication to sobriety. Remember, your routine is adaptable — tailor it to fit your growth and evolving needs.

Celebrate your progress

Every step you take toward emotional wellness deserves recognition. It's important to pause and appreciate your efforts, no matter how small they may seem. Celebrating your achievements encourages self-worth and motivates to continue striving forward. Your journey in sobriety is filled with numerous milestones — each one an opportunity for celebration. Did you get through a challenging conversation without reverting to old habits? That's a mark of tremendous progress. Did you take a moment for yourself when you felt overwhelmed instead of spiraling? Another victory worth recognizing. Each time you choose a healthy coping mechanism over a destructive habit, you build a stronger foundation for your emotional well-being.

Acknowledge these moments; they prove you are on the path to a better you. Setting tangible goals and celebrating when you meet them creates a pattern of positive reinforcement, boosting your confidence and reinforcing the healthy behaviors that contribute to your emotional wellness. Your progress may sometimes be incremental, and that's perfectly okay. Healing and growth often come in waves, and each stride forward signifies a personal evolution, no matter how modest. Your perseverance in the face of challenges, your dedication to bettering yourself, and the conscious decisions you make each day are worth more than just acknowledgment — they are triumphs in their own right.

As you stand today, take a moment to honor your strides toward emotional wellness. These steps, big or small, are milestones on your remarkable sobriety journey. Celebrate every achievement as it comes — each challenging conversation navigated, every overwhelming moment met with calm — it's a testament to your progress. By choosing constructive coping mechanisms, you're laying bricks for a robust foundation of emotional health.

Chapter 9

Finding Your Purpose and Joy

Deciding to live without alcohol long-term is a decision that ushers in a life rich with fresh starts and possibilities for personal rediscovery. Letting go of alcohol and other mind-altering substances enables a clearer perspective on life. You are empowered to shape your story, find *your purpose*, and engage in activities that genuinely excite and fulfill you. This freedom journey allows you to focus on what you genuinely want and cultivate the hobbies, skills, and relationships that align with who you truly are.

In this chapter, we explore the different experiences of being sober. This is not a straightforward path but a rich journey from moments of curiosity and self-discovery. You're encouraged to grant yourself the freedom to experiment with new hobbies and interests, trying things you've always wanted to try, each experience revealing more of who you are and what you love. Sobriety means making your life so awesome and fun that you don't even miss alcohol. It's all about filling up with good stuff that feeds your mind, heart, and soul. As you embark on this new phase, immerse yourself in the activities and passions that bring you joy and celebrate the boundless opportunities. Embrace the richness of your recovery. In doing so, you can build a life so good you will never want to return to drinking.

Exploring Personal Passions and Interests

Before sobriety, your life may have felt dictated by habits and external demands. Now, you can carve your path based on personal passions and intrinsic interests. Stepping off the beaten path and uncovering what ignites your spirit requires bravery and action.

In rediscovering your joy, it's essential to give yourself permission to explore new territories and reinvent your definition of happiness. The things you once enjoyed might not resonate with you anymore, and that's okay. Sobriety opens up a space to explore various hobbies and activities that could bring newfound joy. Embrace the process with an open mind and let curiosity be your guide.

Let's create a sobriety vision board that allows you to visually explore and identify new sources of joy and passion in your sobriety journey.

Materials needed:

>> Magazines

>> Colored paper

>> Scissors

>> Glue

>> Large poster board or cardboard

Follow these instructions:

1. **Set the scene:** Find a comfortable and quiet space to spread out your materials.

2. **Reflect:** Take a few deep breaths and reflect on what brought you joy in the past and what excites you now. Think about areas you haven't explored yet but are curious about. Write a list so you can refer back to it while you search.

3. **Cut and collect:** Flip through magazines or print out images from online sources that resonate with your interests or potential new hobbies. These could include images of nature, art, sports, musical instruments, books, travel destinations, and so on.

4. **Assemble your collage:** Start gluing the images onto your poster board in a visually pleasing way. Don't overthink the process; let it be intuitive and spontaneous.

5. **Personalize:** Use colored paper or markers to add personal touches, such as quotes, affirmations, or specific goals for each image.

6. **Reflect and share:** Once you've completed your collage, step back and reflect on what you see. What themes emerge? Which images make you feel the most excited? If you feel comfortable, share your vision board with a supportive friend, family member, or even a sobriety support group. Discussing your vision board can provide additional insight and encouragement. Make sure you take note of the feedback you receive.

7. **Act on it:** Choose one image that stands out and commit to exploring that interest within the next week. It could be as simple as reading a book on the subject, joining a class, or attending an event.

This creative exercise allows you to tap into your artistic side and visualize a future filled with activities that bring you genuine happiness. It's a physical representation of the joy you're carving out for yourself in this new chapter of your life.

TIP

This is a great exercise to do with like-minded people. Gather a few of your closest friends, set up some appetizers, and have a fun evening of vision board creation.

REMEMBER

It's often the case that society's norms can cloud your perception of what brings pleasure, chaining you to expectations rather than true satisfaction. Sobriety breaks these chains, encouraging you to set out on a journey toward self-discovery. As you travel this road, focus on identifying pastimes that vibrate with excitement for you. Whether it's art, music, nature, or any other endeavor that calls to you — dive in and let that passion fill your life with joy and purpose.

Don't underestimate the power of supportive relationships in this journey. Surround yourself with people encouraging your explorations and inspiring you to reach further. Push through the discomfort of the unfamiliar, and you'll find your people — those special individuals who not only appreciate your newfound interests but may also share them. Relationships are crucial as they provide companionship and reinforce your purpose, multiplying the joy you derive from your passions. These people will give you the space you need to be the best version of yourself.

Identifying hobbies and activities that bring joy

Your journey to joy begins with identifying hobbies and activities that truly resonate with you. These are pursuits that energize rather than drain, that cause hours to pass like minutes. Find your happiness by trying things that make you feel super alive. Whether it's painting, gardening, or walking in the woods, it's essential to let yourself try new stuff. Don't hesitate to leave your comfort zone to discover hobbies that light up your spirit. After all, the most amazing experiences tend to happen outside our comfort zone.

Take the time to reflect on your past experiences and consider the moments you felt most content. Was it when you were crafting something with your hands or perhaps solving a challenging puzzle? Let these memories serve as clues to your passions. Remember, the goal is to engage in activities that bring enthusiasm in your heart. Consider taking a course, joining a club, or simply dedicating a quiet corner of your weekend to indulge in those activities that make you feel happy.

Listen to your body and mood as you dive into these activities. Notice how each hobby influences your emotional and physical state. Are you feeling invigorated after a dance class, or are you left in a state of blissful peace after a meditation session? Pursue these signs of joy. Moreover, these activities aren't just pastimes; they're stepping stones to a deeper understanding of yourself and what brings meaning to your life. They help you make new friends and find groups who like what you like, building friendships that help and support you.

Now, explore your interests to identify hobbies and activities that provide fulfillment and joy in a substance-free lifestyle.

Materials needed:

>> Notebook, paper, or journal

>> A pen or pencil

>> An open mind (essential)

TIP

Using a computer or other electronic device can be less effective. When you write by hand, you activate your brain's Reticular Activation System (RAS), which helps maintain focus and filter relevant information. The RAS acts as a gatekeeper, directing important information to your conscious awareness. It works with other brain regions, like the prefrontal cortex, to enhance your ability to organize thoughts, synthesize information, and make connections between concepts.

Follow these steps:

1. **Make a list:** Begin by listing all the hobbies and activities mentioned in your knowledge base that intrigue you: adventure sports, advanced classes, travel, mentorship, community theater, home improvement projects, horticulture, cooking classes, volunteering, group sports, learning a new language or instrument, and so on.

2. **Research and reflect:** For each listed item, spend some time researching what it entails, how you might get involved, and its benefits. Jot down any thoughts or feelings that arise during this process.

3. **Plan an adventure:** Choose one activity from your list to try out. Plan a simple, low-risk way to explore this hobby. For example, if you're interested in horticulture, visit a local nursery or botanical garden, or if community theater piqued your interest, attend a local performance or audition.

4. **Engage and evaluate:** After engaging in the activity, reflect on the experience. How did it make you feel? Did time fly by? Did it spark joy or provide a sense of achievement? Write down your reflections.

5. **Repeat and expand:** In the spirit of exploration, make it a goal to try out a new activity from your list regularly. As you test different hobbies, some might resonate more than others, guiding you toward what truly brings joy.

6. **Integrate:** Once you find an activity that lights up your spirit, look for ways to integrate it into your routine. Perhaps you could join a club or group related to the hobby or dedicate a specific time each week to indulge in it.

7. **Connect to a community:** Seek out local or online communities that share your newfound interests. Engaging with others can add a social dimension to your hobby and provide additional motivation and support.

Exploring and integrating new hobbies is inspired by various holistic and self-discovery practices advocated in sobriety and personal development literature. The activity is tailored to help you rediscover the joy in your life by methodically seeking out and trying new hobbies, reflecting on the experiences, and consciously choosing to incorporate the ones that bring true happiness into your regular life.

REMEMBER

It's essential also to be patient with the process. Identifying your passions doesn't happen overnight, and your interests may evolve. Remain open-minded and allow yourself the freedom to shift gears. Perhaps an interest that once captivated you no longer sparks the same joy — and that's okay. Give yourself the grace to let go and move forward, continuously seeking out and embracing the countless possibilities that await you. As you embark on this quest for joy and purpose, embrace the journey as much as the destination, savoring each moment of discovery and every milestone of personal achievement.

Reconnecting with long-forgotten interests

Sobriety often introduces new insights and a different way of seeing the world. As you progress in your recovery, you might find yourself reconnecting with interests and pastimes that addiction has pushed aside. These activities, whether they involve creating artwork, making music, reading, or any other pursuit, can offer a profound sense of comfort and fulfillment that may have been elusive. Choosing sobriety every day is like rediscovering a part of yourself that has always been there, preserved, and ready for you to engage with once again. Pick up your guitar, dive back into that unfinished book, or return to your canvas; these passions are an essential aspect of who you are and can play a significant role in your life of sobriety.

Journaling your interests

Finding your interests is a journey of self-discovery that can help you lead a fulfilling and purpose-driven life. It involves exploring various activities, hobbies, and subjects to determine what genuinely excites and motivates you. This process can be both introspective and experiential, requiring you to try new things, reflect on past experiences, and recognize patterns in what you enjoy.

Journaling your interests can be an invaluable tool in this discovery process. By documenting your thoughts, feelings, and reactions to different activities, you can gain deeper insights into what truly engages and satisfies you.

Here are 20 hobby and activity ideas to get you started on reconnecting with long-forgotten interests or discovering new ones in your journey of sobriety. Have you done any of these? What's been your experience with them? Pick up your journal and take some notes on each:

1. **Adventure sports:** Try rock climbing or hiking for a burst of adrenaline.

2. **Yoga or Tai Chi:** Gentle exercise for body-mind harmony.

3. **Art classes:** Dive into painting, drawing, or pottery for creative expression.

4. **Music therapy:** Play instruments or write music to articulate emotions.

5. **Gardening:** Cultivate a garden for tranquility and the satisfaction of growth.

6. **Cooking classes:** Learn new recipes and techniques for healthy living.

7. **Mindfulness and meditation:** For stress management and inner peace.

8. **Volunteering:** Give back to your community and find purpose.

9. **Group sports:** Join a local softball team or bowling league for fun and fitness.

10. **Language lessons:** Challenge your mind and expand your horizons.

11. **Instrument lessons:** Pick up that guitar or sit down at a piano and start playing.

12. **Spiritual retreats:** Explore spirituality and find inner calm.

13. **Adventure sports:** Try rock climbing or hiking for a burst of adrenaline.

14. **Writing:** Journal your journey or start a blog to share your experiences.

15. **Exercise:** Find a physical activity like swimming or cycling.

16. **Book clubs:** Reconnect with literature and meet new people.

17. **Home improvement projects:** Channel creativity into your living space.

18. **Advocacy or activism:** Make a stand on issues you care about.

19. **Art exhibitions or music performances:** Showcase your talents or enjoy others'.

20. **Advanced education:** Enroll in courses that interest you.

Embrace these activities as opportunities for growth and joy in your sober life. They're more than hobbies; they help you discover who you are, connect with others, and really enjoy life's many adventures. Now, start creating a list of your own.

REMEMBER

It's not uncommon for those in recovery to struggle with how to fill their time now that their addiction no longer consumes it. You can turn to those once-loved activities for a sense of purpose and joy. The time you spent in addiction can now be used for creativity and learning. It's a chance to rekindle the excitement of learning, to grow and master new skills, or even just to savor the simple pleasure of doing something for its own sake. These activities bring personal satisfaction and significantly strengthen sobriety by creating positive, fulfilling routines that support your new lifestyle.

Engaging in pastimes connects you with communities of like-minded individuals. Consider the energy and inspiration you can draw from joining a local book club, finding a music group, or participating in an art class. These connections can provide encouragement and companionship, fostering relationships built on common interests rather than shared vices. You may find added motivation and support for your sober journey as you interact with others who share your sober lifestyle. So, grab this chance to explore all the good things sobriety brings. Let your heart guide you toward the interests that resonate with you, and watch as joy and purpose cascade into your new, healthier life.

Channeling creativity as a source of purpose

Creativity is the lifeline that courses through every activity, hobby, or task you undertake. It's more than just painting or making music. It's about the new ideas you bring to dinner, the fun changes you make to a board game, and the smart fixes you find for work problems. Picture your life as a canvas. How do you want to fill it up? By engaging with the world in a way that fuels your uniqueness and offers new perspectives, you create a path to self-discovery. Use this natural ability because it's how many people find their purpose and endless happiness.

Your creative path doesn't have to stick to a set plan. It's a path as individual as a fingerprint, where each choice and contribution amounts to a larger depiction of who you are. Jump into your imagination with excitement; enjoy your intelligent ideas. Whether you turn leftovers into a fancy meal or make a garden from empty land, you're the boss of creating new things. Creativity can manifest in a well-organized spreadsheet's efficiency or a compelling presentation's creativeness, even in your professional life. By facing new challenges and trying new things in all parts of your life, you'll see that being creative is not just a way to have fun — it helps you find happiness and meaning.

REMEMBER

Your creativity is like an endless source waiting to be used. It resonates in how you solve problems, entertain ideas, and interact with the people around you. The world craves your originality, and by nurturing it, you enrich your experiences and contribute in a way that adds value to society. Incorporating creativity into your daily life requires intentionality, choosing to see the special in the everyday. With this thinking, you'll find creative ideas hidden in surprising places, ready to grow when you pay attention and act on them. As you channel your creative energies, take pride in knowing that each spark of creativity brings you closer to recognizing your full potential and finding authentic joy in your existence.

Enjoying Meaningful Connections and Relationships

Finding and holding on to your purpose can help guide you through challenging times. This resilience is anchored in discovering your passions and the meaningful connections and relationships you build. Deep, empathetic bonds with others can serve as a lifeline, providing support and a sense of belonging essential to maintaining sobriety. Investing in relationships that resonate with your true self creates a nurturing environment for personal growth and healing. Remember, you are not meant to walk this journey alone.

Giving back to your community and contributing in ways that align with your values instills a profound sense of purpose. It demonstrates that your existence has relevance beyond your immediate surroundings. Whether through volunteer work, mentorship, or simply offering kindness to strangers, service reinforces the idea that you are a part of something larger than yourself. And remember, this does not necessarily have to be within sober communities; the effects of your positive contributions ripple through all aspects of society.

REMEMBER

Maintaining a balance between nurturing your connections and seeking fulfillment within yourself is super important. While solid relationships can provide support, your happiness should not solely depend on others. Cultivate self-appreciation and set goals that fulfill you personally and professionally. Aligning your objectives with your innate purpose and having intrinsic motivation is key. And as you set these goals, remember to enjoy the journey. Revel in the small steps you take toward them, allowing yourself to find joy rather than fixating solely on the destination.

Building meaningful relationships in sobriety

Building meaningful relationships in sobriety is a transformative and essential component of the journey toward a fulfilling, sober life. When you find yourself on this path, creating and growing bonds with individuals who understand your journey and support and reinforce your commitment to sobriety becomes essential. Have you heard the saying, You are the average of the five people you spend the most time with – a concept often attributed to motivational speaker Jim Rohn. In the early stages of this transition, you usually face reevaluating your current relationships. You might find that some of the connections that seemed significant in the past no longer serve your best interests. It's about seeking out those who resonate with your innermost values and who encourage your passions and pursuits without the influence of substances.

As you continue to evolve in your sobriety, you'll discover that your connections are about quality rather than quantity. It's important to cultivate relationships that provide a sense of joy and purpose rather than those that simply fill your time. This shift in perspective might mean stepping away from relationships predicated on shared habits that no longer fit with your sober life. Instead, you will start attracting and recognizing individuals who appreciate your true self, are interested in your welfare, and will walk alongside you without judgment.

REMEMBER

As you grow, your relationships should reflect that growth, bringing into your life people who are meant for your season, serve a specific reason in your journey, or are meant to stay for a lifetime.

CHEERS TO CHANGE: TOASTING TO SOBRIETY AND AUTHENTICITY WITH TIANA

One of the most complex parts of getting sober was leaving my old life behind. I was under the illusion that the life I once lived was filled with close friendships and fun times. Looking back now, though, I realize it was the exact opposite. Ending an evening in a blackout state and asking questions the following day to figure out who I had to apologize to for my behavior wasn't exactly something I would now classify as fun.

A few months after I had gotten sober, I decided to hold onto some of these old friendships; I would attend a house party one of my friends was hosting. This regular event involved food, booze, and usually a bonfire. Sounds like fun, right? With my six-pack of Diet Coke in hand, I headed over to attempt to fit into a world that created a lot of self-destruction, but this time, I was going to do it sober and be responsible.

When I got to their place, I was greeted with hugs and praises for getting sober. It felt good to have my friends tell me they supported my new lifestyle yet allowed me to continue to be a part of their world. As the afternoon continued, I ran out of Diet Coke quickly. I became very aware that although I wasn't drinking alcohol, the habit of matching people's drink for drink was very much still alive. Why would someone drink a six-pack of Diet Coke in just over an hour? It was because I wanted to fit in. I remember one of my friends noticing someone approaching me with a drink in hand. She quickly ran over and asked them not to go near me with the alcoholic beverage. She was also very drunk, and that action made me feel very uncomfortable. Not to mention the change in conversation as everyone continued to get increasingly drunk; it wasn't real, and it certainly wasn't authentic.

At that moment, I realized this was not where I wanted to be. I didn't want my life to revolve around house parties and pub crawls, and I apologized for the mistakes I made the night before that I had no recollection of. I wanted honest conversations with people who created space and room for personal growth. I tried to listen to someone tell me what they planned to do with their life and know that it was the truth and that they would take action to make that happen.

I got sober through a 12-step program, and although I realize this way of getting sober is not for everyone, it allowed me to build an incredible support network of people who want to be of service to others. It's also taught me to deal with my past so that I could learn from my mistakes and continue to create new opportunities to live a life full of joy and purpose. I have been through many hard times in my life of sobriety, but the people I surround myself with today have made those times easier to move through. They haven't offered me a drink or suggested a night out at the pub so that I could forget my troubles. Instead, they provide a safe space so that I can deal with them in a more healthy way that will create healing and happiness.

REMEMBER

Embracing sobriety is also about relearning to form relationships on a more authentic level. Partnerships in this phase of life need to be built on solid foundations of trust, understanding and shared experiences that don't rely on old socializing habits. Here, meaningful conversations, mutual support, and shared laughter become the currency of your relationships. This rewiring of how you connect with others isn't always easy, but it's enriching. Such connections enhance your daily experience and fortify your resolve to maintain sobriety. Finding your tribe — those unique individuals who add color to the canvas of your life — becomes an adventure in itself, an integral part of living a life aligned with your true purpose and joy.

Contributing to the community and others

Transcending beyond personal gains, contributing to your community and others can imbue your life with a more profound sense of purpose. In sobriety, the act of giving takes on a new significance. It's not solely about offering your time or resources to sober circles; it's about reaching out to any part of your community where you can make a difference — no matter how small it may seem. Discover that when you contribute to the well-being of others without expecting anything in return, the satisfaction derived can be far greater than any material reward.

When you're on the path to finding your purpose, consider how your unique skills and passions can benefit others. Think about what energizes you, and then explore how those activities can intersect with community needs. For example, if you love gardening, you can volunteer at a local park or start a community garden, contributing to neighborhood beautification and communal eating. If teaching is your passion, offer complimentary classes in a subject you know about, helping educate and uplift those around you.

Next, we'll build community connections by identifying ways to contribute to your community that align with your interests and creating an action plan to make a meaningful impact.

Materials needed:

>> A journal or notepad

>> A pen or pencil

>> An electronic device

>> A calendar

>> Internet access if you need to research

Instructions:

1. **Pause for self-reflection:** Take a moment to reflect on your passions and skills. What do you love doing? What are you good at? Write these down in your journal.

2. **Research local needs:** Look into local organizations, nonprofits, and community groups. What needs in your community resonate with you? Make a list of these needs alongside your identified passions and skills.

3. **Find at least three exciting ideas:** Using your journal, brainstorm ways to bridge the gap between what you love doing and your community's needs. Aim to come up with at least three ideas that excite you. For example, if you enjoy gardening and your community has a local garden that needs tending, you could volunteer to help maintain it and share your expertise.

4. **Create a plan:** Choose one of your ideas to implement first. Outline the steps you need to take to get started. This might include contacting organizations, sourcing materials, or scheduling time to work on your project.

5. **Set SMART (specific, measurable, achievable, relevant, and time-bound) goals:** Setting goals for your chosen activity helps ensure you follow through. Write these down in your journal.

6. **Take action:** Take the first step outlined in your plan. This could be as simple as sending an email to a local charity or as involved as attending a community meeting.

7. **Build relationships:** As you engage in your chosen activity, consciously connect with the people involved. Share your journey of sobriety only if you feel comfortable, and focus on building supportive, meaningful relationships.

8. **Reflect and adjust:** After you have started your activity, regularly reflect on your experiences. How does contributing make you feel? What have you learned? Adjust your plan as needed, and if you feel called to, explore additional ways to contribute.

9. **Celebrate and share:** Celebrate your contributions, no matter how small, and consider sharing your experiences with others in your sober circle or support group. This can inspire others and strengthen your commitment to your sober journey.

This exercise isn't about overwhelming yourself with commitments but finding joy and purpose in contributing to the community that aligns with your interests and supports your sobriety.

REMEMBER

Investing in your community isn't just about the output of your efforts; it's also about the relationships you build along the way. These connections can support, encourage growth, and foster a sense of belonging — critical elements in maintaining sobriety and finding joy. As you give to your community, you'll likely find that you're not just changing others' lives but profoundly impacting your own. Helping can reinforce your sense of purpose, solidify your sobriety, and ultimately lead to a more fulfilling and joyous existence.

Balancing social connections for personal fulfillment

Balancing social connections is essential for your fulfillment in sobriety. Cherish the times of solitude, appreciating the peace they can bring without letting them spiral into loneliness. Simultaneously, participate in social activities that resonate with your passions, ensuring you do not deplete yourself by overcommitting. It's all about fostering relationships that increase your self-esteem and make you feel valued for who you are — not for the unrealistic expectations others may place.

Your long-term sober journey is unique, which means setting boundaries for self-care where necessary while also being open to widening your circle of friends and acquaintances to benefit from various perspectives and support systems. One of the most powerful words you can use in sobriety is no. This balance is critical to lasting happiness and feeling purposeful as you live soberly. By doing so, you actively create an environment conducive to your personal growth and emotional health.

REMEMBER

The quality of your relationships often matters more than the quantity. Invest in connections that encourage mutual growth and understanding. Seek out those who uplift you and recognize when moving on from relationships that no longer serve your well-being is healthy. The art of balance is not static — it's an active, ongoing process. It requires attentiveness and adjustments to maintain rhythm and flow like a dance. Embrace this process with a gentle but firm resolve, and find your stride in the rich tapestry of interconnected human experiences that shape a fulfilling, sober life.

Setting and Pursuing Life Goals

Understanding the gravity of setting and pursuing life goals is pivotal in your journey toward long-term sobriety and personal fulfillment. It's a process that requires deep introspection and a willingness to align your actions with your core values and interests. Imagine guiding your life's journey across an expansive field of opportunities, plotting a path that reflects your unique essence; this is the heart of setting your life goals. It's not just about hitting society's goals or copying others' success. It's about creating a dream that excites you every day.

Life goals should be like a compass, guiding your steps with purpose and intention. When you set goals that reflect who you truly are and what you genuinely desire, you create a roadmap for a life filled with intrinsic motivation. Your goals shouldn't be static, unchangeable end-points but rather evolving landmarks that move and grow as you do. Focus on the process of achieving a goal and not the outcome; you will enjoy it more that way. This fluid approach ensures that the weight of unmet expectations does not crush you but is uplifted by each achievement, no matter how small. Enjoy the journey and celebrate small wins because these moments make up a happy life.

Discover your Ikigai

Discovering your Ikigai — the Japanese concept of finding one's reason for being — can be a transformative step in your sober journey. It offers a profound sense of purpose that aligns with your passions, talents, and the world's needs.

In this exercise, we will explore your inner landscape and identify your Ikigai, a converging point of what you love, what you are good at, what the world needs, and what you can be rewarded for.

Materials needed:

>> Four sheets of paper

>> A pen or pencil

>> A comfortable, quiet space

>> Optionally, an Ikigai diagram template

Follow these instructions:

1. **Prepare your space:** Find a quiet space where you won't be interrupted. This exercise requires introspection and honesty with yourself.

2. **Find what you love (your passion):** On the first sheet of paper, answer this question: What activities make you feel excited and passionate? In other words, what do you absolutely love doing in your free time? These should be things that you enjoy so much that time seems to fly by when you're doing them.

3. **Discover what you are good at (your vocation):** On the second sheet of paper, reflect on your skills and strengths. What tasks do you find easy? What do people often compliment you about or seek your help with?

TIP

If you're struggling to develop ideas about your skills, text three to five people you trust and ask, "If you could come to me for advice on anything, what would that be? What do you think are my strengths?"

4. **Identify what the world needs (your mission):** On the third sheet of paper, ponder on the needs of the world that resonate with you. What issues or causes do you feel strongly about? Think about what you believe would make the world a better place.

5. **Zero in on what you can be rewarded for (your profession):** On the fourth sheet of paper, consider what services or contributions you can offer that others would be willing to pay for. What skills or knowledge do you have that are in demand?

6. **Find the intersections:** Place the four sheets of paper out in front of you and start looking for commonalities. Your Ikigai resides where these four elements intersect. It's the sweet spot that incorporates what you love, what you are good at, what the world needs, and what you can be paid for.

7. **Draw your Ikigai diagram (optional):** If you're a visual person, drawing an Ikigai diagram can help you visualize the overlap between these four areas. Sketch four overlapping circles, each representing one of the elements, with a space in the center for your Ikigai. See Figure 9-1 for an example.

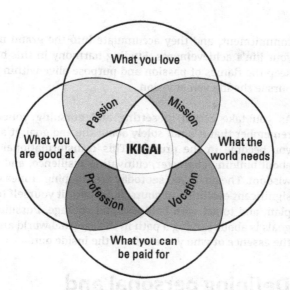

FIGURE 9-1:
Ikigai.

Within the figure:
What you love

Passion

Mission

What you are good at

IKIGAI

What the world needs

Profession

Vocation

What you can be paid for

8. **Reflect and synthesize:** Reflect on the intersections you've identified. What insight can you draw from them? Begin to synthesize these into a coherent statement of your Ikigai.

9. **Create an action plan:** With your Ikigai in mind, consider how to incorporate it into your daily life. What small steps can you take to start living in alignment with your Ikigai? Set realistic goals and a timeline to achieve them.

10. **Review and adapt:** Life is dynamic, and so is your Ikigai. Periodically revisit your Ikigai and the steps you're taking to embody it. Make adjustments as needed, and celebrate the progress you make along the way.

This activity is about self-discovery and creating a sustainable lifestyle that fuels your sobriety with meaning and joy. Finding your Ikigai is a journey, not a destination, so be kind to yourself throughout the process.

Balancing aspiration with realism is critical as you set your personal and professional goals. Aim high, but plant your ladder firmly based on your capabilities and circumstances. It's important to challenge yourself, but equally vital to recognize and embrace your limits to avoid burnout and disillusionment. As you tread the path toward your goals, celebrate the small victories. Each tiny win is a testament to your perseverance and commitment, and they accumulate into the grand narrative of your life's achievements. Finding harmony in this balance will keep the flames of passion and purpose alive within you as you pursue the life you envision.

REMEMBER

As you take action in setting and pursuing your life goals, remember that it's not solely about the end goal; it's about who you become in the process. This transformational journey is about building character, cultivating resilience, and growing in wisdom. The goals you set today are stepping stones to the more significant evolution of yourself. So permit yourself to dream, to plan, and to act with boldness and courage. Pursuing your life goals is about carving a path in the external world and sculpting the essence of who you are from the inside out.

Defining personal and professional aspirations

Your journey toward joy and purpose is not just a pursuit; it's a discovery. You must explore yourself to truly find what sets your heart alight and gives your life a deeply rooted meaning. Start by pinpointing precisely what makes you tick — those activities, ideas, and dreams that surge through you with enthusiasm. What excites you? What projects, hobbies, or causes do you find immersive to the point of losing track of time? Within these moments, your purpose may be whispering to you, coaxing you to bring those passions into the light and integrate them into your daily life. Having a sense of purpose can give you additional intrinsic motivation to overcome sobriety challenges.

Your professional aspirations are equally important and should be more than just financial milestones. They should align with your innermost convictions, allowing you to pursue a career that's both successful and fulfilling. Ask yourself, are you following a path you've chosen or one laid out for you by others? To make your professional journey rewarding, your career should tap into your skill set and resonate with your personal beliefs and values. Here, your profession meets your passion, transforming what you do into a testament to who you are. This alignment breathes life into your work, making every achievement a personal and professional triumph.

Consider the Japanese concept of Ikigai we did earlier in the chapter which encapsulates the essence of life's worth. (If you skipped this, be sure to go back and work through it because it will be worth it.) It offers a blueprint for balance, uniting what you excel at with what you adore doing, all while making sure the world benefits too and also providing you a living. This search for harmony is a fine balancing act; it takes patience and introspection. Take stock of what you contribute to the world and how you can turn it into a vocation. Pursuing your Ikigai isn't about finding perfection but about striving for congruence, where your life's work becomes a reflection of your true self, and in that reflection, you find joy.

Creating realistic and achievable goals

As you venture through the journey of sobriety and personal growth, it's crucial to set goals that are inspiring and grounded in reality. This balance is fundamental in fostering progress without setting yourself up for potential discouragement. Picture your larger aspirations as a series of steps rather than a giant leap. Each step represents a smaller, achievable target that propels you closer to your ultimate ambition. By approaching your dreams incrementally, you make them more attainable and allow yourself the gratification of celebrating each success along the way. This process generates momentum, sustains motivation, and imbues your path with a sense of direction.

Now, let's deconstruct your main goal into manageable, achievable milestones that will guide your progress throughout the year.

Materials needed:

>> A journal, notepad, or electronic device

>> A pen or pencil

>> A quiet space for contemplation

Follow these instructions:

1. **Define your main goal:** Write down your overarching goal. This should be a significant aspiration that you wish to achieve that resonates deeply with your desires and values.

2. **Understand the why:** Reflect on why this goal is important to you. Understanding the underlying motivation will serve as a compass, keeping you directed and energized when challenges arise.

3. **Brainstorm:** Jot down all the tasks you think are necessary to achieve your main goal, no matter how big or small. Don't worry about organizing them yet; just get your ideas on paper.

4. **Categorize and sequence:** Look at the tasks you've listed and group them into categories based on similarity or sequence. Then, arrange these categories into a logical order that builds from one step to the next.

5. **Create 12 milestones:** Divide these categories and tasks into 12 milestones, each representing a step toward your main goal. Each one should be significant enough to feel like progress but also realistic for you to accomplish within a month or a designated time frame.

6. **Detail each milestone:** Write a clear and concise description for each of the 12 milestones. Ensure that each step is actionable and measurable — you should be able to clearly define when it's been achieved.

7. **Set mini-goals:** Within each milestone, set smaller goals or tasks that must be completed. These mini-goals can often be achieved in a day or a week, providing a clear path forward.

8. **Create a timeline:** Assign each milestone a month or a specific timeframe. This will help you stay on track and keep the pace needed to reach your main goal within your desired period.

9. **Be flexible:** Review your milestones and mini-goals to ensure flexibility. Life can be unpredictable, so building in the possibility for adjustments is crucial for maintaining progress.

10. **Start with milestone one:** Focus on the first milestone only. Break down its mini-goals into weekly or even daily tasks and start working on them. This helps prevent feeling overwhelmed by the entire task ahead.

11. **Reflect and adapt:** At the end of each month or timeframe, reflect on the milestone you've worked toward. Celebrate your success, evaluate what worked and what didn't, and adjust your plan for the next milestone accordingly.

12. **Reassess goals:** Periodically, reassess your main goal and the remaining milestones. Are they still relevant and serving your purpose? Don't be afraid to adjust or even change your goal to suit your evolving self better.

REMEMBER

The key to this exercise isn't speed; it's consistent, considered progress. Each step you complete is a win; over time, these successes will accumulate into achieving your main goal. Celebrate each milestone, no matter how small, as a testament to your commitment to your sobriety and personal growth.

REMEMBER

Your life's narrative will undoubtedly twist and turn, and your goals should fluidly adapt to these changes. Rigidity or a fixed mindset can lead to frustration, but with a flexible mindset, you'll navigate the ebb and flow of life with resilience. Encountering new experiences and evolving interests might shift your priorities, and that's perfectly okay. Goals are not set in stone; they are living aspirations that grow and change as you do. Moreover, should a goal no longer serve your purpose or bring joy, you can alter or abandon it in favor of something more aligned with your current self.

Celebrating each small victory, you learn to savor the personal development journey instead of being singularly fixated on the destination. This approach helps you to appreciate the richness of your experiences, acknowledging that fulfillment often resides in the steps toward achieving your ambitions. By taking time to rejoice in incremental progress, you establish a practice of gratitude and mindfulness that enhances your overall well-being. Remember, your journey toward your goals is as significant as the goals themselves, as it shapes who you become while striving toward them.

4

Overcoming Challenges and Thriving in Sobriety

Chapter **10**

Handling Challenges and Relapse

I n the journey of living alcohol-free, you'll encounter certain moments or situations that prod at your resolve, tempting you to fall back into old drinking and using behaviors. These moments, commonly known as *triggers*, are stimuli that *spark* an emotional or physical response, often leading to a craving. To foster a more constructive dialogue around this concept, let's refer to them as *spark points*. Spark points are unique to each individual and can arise from stress, particular memories, or even sensory experiences like sights and smells that were once associated with alcohol. Recognizing your *personal* spark points is a critical step in fortifying your commitment to sobriety and charting a sustainable path forward.

This goes beyond identifying your spark points; it's about mastering your responses to them — sharpening your emotional expression from broad feelings to targeted strategies.

We will uncover a range of approaches to reinforcing your sobriety, which could entail environmental tweaks or reliance on your support network. You'll compile a toolkit of coping skills to navigate challenges, essential for fostering self-awareness, resilience, and a steadfast alcohol-free commitment.

In this chapter, we will dissect various spark points and equip you with analytical tools to understand your unique experiences with them through emotional triggers, social scenarios, or daily alcohol-related reminders.

Recognizing and Understanding Triggers (aka Sparks)

As you continue to walk on your path to long-term sobriety, it's essential to acknowledge the moments or situations that can challenge your resolve, which we'll refer to as *spark points*, others may call them *triggers*. These are silent alarms that can quietly undermine your progress and potentially ignite a relapse if not managed properly. Determining and addressing these spark points is crucial for flourishing in your alcohol-free life.

Spark points vary widely, and comprehending your personal set is crucial in sustaining sobriety. Emotional spark points, such as stress, anxiety, and even seemingly positive emotions like excitement, can unexpectedly lead to cravings. Environmental factors count, too; having alcohol in your home or visiting past drinking haunts can stir up old patterns. It demands deliberate effort to cultivate a sober-friendly space and to nurture the emotional resilience needed to handle these spark points.

To better manage these spark points, actively engage with your emotions and articulate them. This might be a bit awkward at the beginning, but recognizing your emotions empowers you to confront them. Using "I" statements is beneficial here; by expressing "I feel stressed in this scenario," you gain more clarity and command over the situation. Plus, drawing on your community for support, whether through friends, family, or support groups, can act as a lifeline during overwhelming moments.

There's immense value in having a diverse array of coping strategies. Mindfulness techniques, balanced nutrition, and stress relief methods are invaluable resources. Your journey will likely require different approaches at various points, and that's absolutely okay. The key is to have a set of tools at the ready to help you steer through the challenges associated with spark points and the risk of relapse.

Mapping your spark points

Regularly journal your spark points to swiftly recognize and defuse them, transforming potential setbacks into stepping stones for your sobriety journey and navigating your journey to long-term sobriety with greater awareness and control.

Let's begin!

1. **Reflect on your spark points:** Take a moment to reflect on times when you felt an urge related to alcohol. What were you doing? Who were you with? What emotions were you feeling?

2. **Create your spark point map:** Draw a large circle on a piece of paper or a digital note-taking app. Divide the circle into segments, like a pie chart, labeling each with different aspects of your life (such as Work, Relationships, Alone Time, Social Events).

3. **Fill in the details:** For each segment, jot down specific instances or feelings that have acted as spark points in the past.

4. **Color code your map:** Use colors to indicate the intensity of each spark point, such as red for high risk, yellow for moderate risk, and green for low risk.

5. **Plan your strategies:** Next to each spark point, write a coping strategy that you could use to handle that particular challenge. If you're unsure, leave it blank for now — you'll fill it in as you learn more strategies.

6. **Find a community connection:** If you're comfortable, discuss your spark point map with a trusted friend, family member, or support group. They can help you brainstorm coping strategies and offer support.

7. **Review and revise:** Keep your map somewhere accessible. As you progress in your sobriety, return to it regularly to update or add new spark points and strategies.

Remember, this map is a living document of your sobriety journey. It will evolve just as you do, becoming an invaluable guide to a fulfilling, alcohol-free life. Stay encouraged; you're not just charting spark points, you're mapping out your success!

Identifying personal emotions for relapse

Walking a path of recovery and understanding the interplay between emotions, depression, and relapse is crucial. This intricate relationship is well-documented in scientific literature as emotional dysregulation. It is a known risk factor for relapse among individuals in recovery from alcoholism and addiction.

Supported by multiple studies, it assures that negative emotional states, particularly depression, can trigger cravings and substance-seeking behaviors. This is due in part to the disruptions that substance use inflicts upon the brain's reward and stress-regulation systems. When an individual's ability to regulate emotional states is compromised, the temptation to return to substance use as a form of self-medication becomes increasingly alluring.

Earlier in this book, we examined the importance of recognizing and managing one's emotional landscape as a critical element in avoiding relapse. Here, the concept of *emotional sobriety* comes into play — a term that encapsulates the ability to experience, *tolerate*, and express emotions effectively.

TIP

Make it a daily practice to tune in to your emotional state with a simple "emotional check-in." Set aside a moment each day to reflect on your feelings and the emotions you're experiencing. This practice can help you recognize early signs of emotional dysregulation or creeping depression. By promptly acknowledging and addressing these feelings, you can reduce the risk of them escalating into *sparks* that could challenge your recovery journey. Remember the core principles of emotional sobriety: experiencing your emotions without judgment, tolerating the discomfort they may bring, and being able to express them healthily. By doing so, you'll actively reinforce your emotional resilience and commitment to long-term sobriety.

As you solidify your recovery groundwork, it's vital to recognize how depression can significantly influence the risk of slipping back into old habits. Studies highlight the critical link between depressive states and the temptation to relapse. These low moods can cast long shadows over our sense of hope and shake our confidence in handling the day-to-day struggles that come with staying sober. However, there are rays of light that can break through this darkness. Regular physical activity, for instance, can lift spirits and build mental toughness, and cultivating a mindset of gratitude can help keep depressive thoughts at bay. Additionally, as we move further away from substance use, our brains have a remarkable ability to heal and rewire themselves, gradually improving our mood and emotional strength. By including these positive actions and attitudes in our recovery plan, we can better safeguard our sobriety against the potential pitfalls of depression.

Additionally, support groups and therapy sessions offer invaluable support for you to explore your emotional states, confront depression, and develop healthier coping strategies. These interventions reinforce new neural pathways in the brain, leading to improved emotional regulation and a more robust defense against the impulse to relapse.

When you focus on nurturing mental wellness in sobriety, we can help those in recovery to combat depression effectively. This includes a holistic approach encompassing mindfulness practices, nutritional considerations, and the maintenance of a balanced daily routine, as discussed in the respective chapters addressing these practices.

Later in this book, we will investigate strategies that can safeguard against depression's detrimental impact on your journey to long-term sobriety.

Anchor your recovery in positive habits

Recall that depression can act like quicksand on the path of recovery, subtly pulling you toward old patterns. It's crucial to stay vigilant about how these emotional undercurrents might affect you. As you work on strengthening your foundation, don't lose sight of the power of positive habits to keep you grounded. Engage in regular exercise to bolster your mood and resilience, and nurture a grateful mindset to fend off negative thoughts.

Tools for emotional navigation

>> **Mindfulness-based stress reduction (MBSR):** Mindfulness teaches you to observe your thoughts and emotions without judgment, helping you to recognize the signs of depression and address them constructively. We talk more about this in Chapter 15.

>> **Ancestral narrative exploration:** By reflecting on your family history, we can gain insights into inherited emotional patterns and how they influence our recovery journey.

>> **Nutritional practices:** Your diet can impact your emotional state. Nutrient-dense foods, for example, can help stabilize mood swings that might otherwise lead to relapse. Refer to Chapter 8 and review Chapter 15.

>> **Daily routines:** A consistent wake-up and bedtime routine can promote better sleep, which is crucial for your emotional and mental health.

Coping with the tides of emotion

As you develop coping mechanisms, you also learn the art of resilience. The ability to return to a state of emotional equilibrium after a depressive episode or emotional upheaval is a sign of actual growth in recovery. You must embrace vulnerability as a strength and recognize that every emotional challenge allows for more profound healing and sobriety reinforcement.

Remember, depression is neither a sign of failure nor a life sentence. It's a signal, an invitation to engage more deeply with your recovery and the community around you. Your emotions hold powerful insights; learning to understand and harness them, can forge a more resilient and joyful path in your long-term recovery.

Environmental and emotional triggers (sparks)

Your immediate environment is a powerful influencer on your behavior and state of mind. It can foster your growth or impede your progress, especially during recovery. An environment that holds reminders of past indulgences, such as keeping alcohol at home, poses a considerable risk of relapse. To combat this, you must re-evaluate your surroundings and remove any items that may cause temptations. Instead, fill your space with positivity and tranquility – include elements that soothe the senses, like peaceful music, delicious food, great-tasting beverages, and even a few plants that can add life and freshness to the room. Making these changes can create a physical barrier against relapse and empower you to maintain your commitment to sobriety.

Your emotional landscape is equally critical in managing your emotions. Emotional triggers such as stress, anxiety, family problems, jealousy, or the weight of isolation can all chip away at your resolve. Acknowledging these triggers and understanding your reactions to them creates an opportunity for change and growth. Developing healthy coping mechanisms — such as journaling, seeking professional counseling, or practicing mindfulness — can help you navigate through these emotional storms without turning to substances as an escape. Remember, recognizing and diffusing these emotional charges is not a sign of weakness; it is an act of strength and a testament to your dedication to your recovery.

Lastly, combining a supportive environment with emotional resilience is crucial for long-term success. Fostering a space where you can freely express emotions and seek solace when needed, surrounded by individuals who care and support your journey, enhances your ability to stand firm against environmental and emotional triggers. Engage in community support groups, connect with others on the same path, and be open to using community resources to uphold your recovery. Every step to bolster your emotional defenses and reinvent your environment brings you closer to a relapse-resistant lifestyle, so take these steps with conviction and a clear vision of your desired future.

Transform your space, transform your recovery

TIP

Consciously curate your environment to safeguard your recovery. A space cluttered with reminders of past habits can be a silent adversary. Take charge by removing temptations and reinventing your surroundings to reflect tranquility and positivity. Integrate elements that engage your senses and bring peace. This proactive approach lays down a tangible barrier to relapse and solidifies your commitment to sobriety. Tend to your emotional environment with equal care, identifying triggers like stress or isolation and countering them with healthy coping strategies like journaling or mindfulness.

Potential relapse rriggers (sparks)

Here is a list designed to serve as a tool for reflection and preparation. By familiarizing yourself with the various environmental, emotional, and physical triggers, you can begin to recognize the specific factors that may challenge your sobriety. The key is identifying these sparks and creating personalized strategies that address each one. As you read through the list, take note of any that resonate with you and consider how you might respond proactively to maintain your hard-won recovery. This awareness and preparation are your safeguards, enabling you to navigate the complexities of life in long-term recovery with confidence and resilience.

Environmental:

>> Alcohol or substance presence in the home

>> Frequenting places where you previously used substances

>> Socializing with individuals who use substances

>> Drug paraphernalia or reminders in your environment

>> Unstructured time or lack of routine

>> Exposure to substance-related content in media

>> Environments where stress is high (such as certain workplaces or social settings)

>> Holiday settings

>> Airports and traveling

Emotional:

>> Stress from work, relationships, or finances

>> Anxiety or panic attacks

>> Boredom or lack of engagement

>> Feelings of depression or hopelessness

>> Loneliness or social isolation

>> Anger or frustration

>> Emotional distress from unresolved traumas

>> Excessive celebration or positive emotions

>> Family interactions and holidays

>> Death of a loved one, family, friend, animal, and so on

Physical:

>> Physical pain or discomfort

>> Withdrawal symptoms or cravings

>> Fatigue or lack of sleep

>> Being in a state of hunger or poor nutrition

>> Sensory cues, such as smells or tastes associated with past substance use

>> Illness or feeling unwell

>> Insufficient physical activity or exercise

>> Female hormone and menstrual cycle

REMEMBER

Identifying your sparks is just the beginning. Developing strategies to manage them is crucial for sustained recovery. We suggest having a plan for responding when you encounter such a moment. This could include reaching out to a support person, engaging in a healthy activity, or practicing mindfulness and relaxation techniques. Understanding these sparks' role in your life empowers you to maintain control over your recovery journey.

Developing strategies to navigate triggers

Navigating through the minefield of triggers that life scatters on your path requires a personalized approach that suits your unique circumstances and challenges. Mindfulness, an often-heralded yet sometimes misunderstood practice, is a pillar in this strategy. Incorporating moments of mindfulness into your daily rhythm allows you to anchor yourself in the present, observing potential triggers with detachment rather than becoming trapped by them. It's about building a mental resilience that empowers you to acknowledge your emotions and thoughts without letting them dictate your actions.

Your physical well-being, supported by a proper diet, is crucial in mitigating the power of triggers. Foods that stabilize your mood and energy levels create a physiological buffer against stress and anxiety, common precursors to relapse. Picture your diet as a steady foundation on which your recovery is built; with every healthful meal, you're reinforcing that foundation, giving yourself a fighting chance against the lure of old habits.

Stress reduction techniques are another essential component in your arsenal for dealing with triggers. Techniques such as deep breathing, progressive muscle relaxation, or engaging in activities that bring you joy can act as safe harbors in times of turmoil. By actively reducing stress, you effectively diminish the impact of triggers, softening their ability to push you toward a relapse. Remember, these are not just one-off measures but daily practices that sculpt a more resilient and sober you over time.

Resilience in the face of setbacks is not inborn; it is cultivated by embracing the idea that a relapse is not the end of the road but rather an opportunity to learn and strengthen your prevention strategies. Seeking support from friends, family, or community resources during these times is not a sign of weakness but a brave step toward lasting recovery. By employing these strategies and surrounding yourself with a support network, you transform potential stumbling blocks into stepping stones for personal growth and sobriety.

REMEMBER

As you navigate living life on life's terms, integrate mindfulness to remain anchored in the present, recognizing potential challenges without succumbing to them. Support your physical resilience with a nourishing diet that stabilizes mood and energy, creating a protective barrier against relapse. Embrace stress-reducing practices and reach out for support, transforming each stumbling block into an opportunity for growth and reinforcing your journey to lasting sobriety.

Coping Mechanisms in Times of Difficulty

In your journey of sobriety, you'll encounter challenges that test your determination, edging you close to relapse. These challenges should be viewed not as defeats but as teachable moments reinforcing your dedication to sober living. Among your crucial coping strategies is mindfulness, which centers on embracing the present moment with full attention. Grounding techniques focusing on your breath or body sensations can serve as anchors, helping you disengage from turmoil and maintain your sobriety.

Effective communication is another cornerstone of handling difficulties. When confronted with situations requiring you to assert your boundaries or express your needs, using "I" statements becomes pivotal. This approach is about taking ownership of your feelings and experiences without placing blame or creating defensiveness in others. For instance, saying, "I feel overwhelmed when we argue like this, and I need a moment to collect my thoughts," is a clear, non-confrontational way of communicating that can defuse tension and facilitate understanding between all parties involved.

Lastly, your circle of support — friends, family, support groups, or professional resources — plays a crucial role during trying times. These networks offer a sense of belonging and connection, reminding you that you are not alone on this journey. Remember, it's not a sign of weakness to reach out and lean on others; it's an act of strength. Sharing your struggles and seeking advice from those who have walked in your shoes can provide new perspectives and reinforce your commitment to sobriety. By embracing these coping mechanisms and developing a relapse prevention plan, you can transform difficulties into moments of empowerment and personal growth.

TIP

Embrace the present and utilize breathwork or sensory awareness to stay centered. Complement this with clear, assertive communication using "I" statements, taking responsibility for your emotions and needs in a way that fosters understanding, not conflict. Never underestimate the strength of your support network; these connections are invaluable in reminding you that you're not alone and can offer fresh insights and encouragement to bolster your resolve to remain sober. Together, these mechanisms create a robust defense against relapse, turning potential setbacks into opportunities for personal fortification.

Mindfulness and stress reduction techniques

When waves of stress threaten to capsize your sobriety boat, anchoring yourself in the present moment can be a lifeline. Practicing mindfulness creates a space between you and your reactions, allowing you to view your situation with clarity and composure. Techniques such as deep breathing, meditation, and progressive muscle relaxation can serve as calming ports in the storm, reducing the impact of anxiety and stress. A proper diet, regular exercise, and adequate sleep are equally important, forming a triad of physical wellness that upholds mental strength. Embracing these practices every day ensures that you fortify your mind and body, readying yourself to meet challenges with equanimity. For a deeper exploration of mindfulness and its profound benefits on your recovery journey, turn to

Chapter 15, where we uncover practices that can elevate your ability to navigate storms gracefully.

Effective communication during challenges

Conflict and disagreement are natural parts of human interaction, but for someone in recovery, they carry the weight of potential triggers. The secret to managing these situations is to avoid them and engage with them through effective communication. Embracing '"I" statements help you convey your emotions honestly while minimizing the risk of triggering defensive reactions. It's essential not just to talk but to listen actively, which involves giving full attention to the speaker, acknowledging their points, and providing feedback that shows understanding and respect.

In the heat of conflict, take a moment to center yourself, remember your communication tools, and proceed with a cool head. Asserting your boundaries is not just about being heard but also about respecting yourself and your recovery journey. Seeking to understand before being understood lays the groundwork for resolving issues without compromising your sobriety.

REMEMBER

Through mindful communication, you navigate conflicts more effectively and build stronger, more supportive relationships. These relationships can become a vital part of your support system, acting as a buffer against the pressures that threaten your sobriety. So, when you find yourself amidst conflict, pause, communicate with intention, listen with empathy, and remember that every conversation is an opportunity to reinforce your commitment to your recovery journey.

Learning and Growing from Relapse Experiences

Relapse may feel like a significant setback in your pursuit of sustained sobriety. Yet, it's imperative to recognize it not as a collapse but as an educational chapter in your recovery narrative. What's often misunderstood is that relapse is a process, not a singular event, with the act of picking up a substance *being the final stage*, not the beginning. This process can be marked by emotional and mental shifts long before any physical substance use occurs.

The most effective intervention can occur in the earlier stages. By learning to identify the warning signs — such as changes in thoughts, feelings, and behaviors — you can take proactive steps to reaffirm your recovery goals. Developing a strong prevention plan, which includes coping skills and a supportive network, is crucial.

Every moment of vulnerability is an opportunity for growth and learning. By dissecting the lead-up to the relapse, you can strengthen your defenses for the future. With each challenge comes the potential to deepen your understanding of your triggers, refine your strategies, and solidify your commitment to sobriety, emerging not weakened but fortified by experience.

Relapse happens. Following are some indications a relapse might occur:

>> **Emotional changes:** Increased anxiety, irritability, or other negative emotional states that are not directly related to substance use.

>> **Mental shifts:** Thinking less rationally, glamorizing past use, or beginning to entertain the idea of using again.

>> **Social disengagement:** Withdrawing from support networks, skipping meetings, or isolating oneself from friends and family who support your recovery.

>> **Behavioral changes:** Neglecting self-care practices, routines, and responsibilities that support sober living.

>> **Loss of structure:** Abandoning the daily schedule and structure that reinforces sobriety, leading to a sense of aimlessness.

>> **Coping strategy breakdown:** Decreased use of or disregarding coping mechanisms that help manage triggers and stress.

>> **Rationalization:** Convincing oneself that using would be manageable or justified under current circumstances.

>> **Planning for use:** Starting to think about when, where, and how to use again, sometimes even making arrangements to access substances.

>> **Actual substance use:** The final stage of relapse is when one consumes alcohol or drugs, completing the relapse process.

REMEMBER

Recognizing these stages as they unfold can empower you to intervene and return to the path of recovery before reaching the point of physical relapse.

Understanding the root causes of relapse

Identifying the root causes of relapse is the first critical step to moving forward after a setback. You may examine the internal and external triggers contributing to your urge to revert to old habits. These triggers can be emotional, such as feeling overwhelmed by stress or anxiety, or environmental, like the presence of alcohol at home or social pressures.

By being aware of these triggers, you can actively work to neutralize them. Engaging in mindfulness practices and creating a calm environment are proactive measures that can substantially decrease the intensity of a trigger. Understanding your own psychological and emotional landscape is not merely insightful — it is empowering, setting the stage for a tailored approach to prevention and recovery.

BUDDING WITH DR. SARAH

During my four decades of sustained sobriety, I've observed countless individuals experience relapses. Some find their way back to recovery; tragically, others do not. The timing of a relapse varies widely; it can happen after months or even decades of abstinence. It's vital to recognize the often subconscious impulses that propel one toward substance use again if one is to succeed in long-term recovery. The term *unconscious drive* is deliberate because many who relapse can't pinpoint the cause.

(continued)

(continued)

Early in my sobriety, professionals referred to a phenomenon known as "budding," an acronym for Building Up to Drink or Drug. Another common adage was, "The relapse happens way before the relapse happens." Our peers could sometimes see us spiraling toward relapse before we acknowledged it ourselves. Signs included agitation, irritability, isolation, euphoria, depression, avoidance, detachment from support systems, overconfidence, claiming to have all the answers, shifting blame, idealizing past substance use, and a host of other negative emotional states. Suddenly, you crave excitement, you're bored, or you seek an escape. We are like relief-seeking missiles; discomfort is our nemesis.

A critical recovery skill is learning to tolerate our mind and body sensations. We used to check out to avoid facing reality — life's inherent discomfort. Recovery means addressing unresolved issues from our past and learning to manage present life situations. After spending so much time numbing ourselves, denying our feelings, and fleeing from our internal worlds, becoming acquainted with our inner selves takes effort. Even sitting quietly for a few minutes can be challenging initially or even for those well into their sobriety. Becoming comfortable with the ebb and flow of our emotions and accepting uncomfortable or negative thoughts is essential for embracing life's inevitable changes.

I've known many who simply transitioned from one addiction to another, avoiding the turmoil boiling beneath the surface — this is known as substitution. Whether it's food, gambling, shopping, technology, video games, relationships, or sex, these diversions shield us from past pain, present stress, or future fears. A friend with 15 years of recovery turned to gambling as an escape. Upon reflection, she understood that she was combating underlying feelings of loneliness, boredom, and unresolved anger from past abuse.

To circumvent these emotions, our brain starts to rationalize, minimize, or deny the severity of the addictive behavior. Thoughts like, "I've earned a break," "It's not as bad as drinking," or "Who am I hurting by indulging in online shopping all day?" arise. Our cognitive processes strive to justify these behaviors, enabling the continuation of addictive patterns.

During graduate school, I recall craving a drink at the end of each semester after the final exams. The residual stress left my body tense, seeking release, and my mind would wander to thoughts of alcohol despite years of abstinence — the addiction's tenacious grip.

One of my patients experienced a pattern of cravings and relapsed every six months. It became clear that by the six-month mark, she could no longer distract herself from the anger stemming from her abusive relationship. Instead of confronting her rage, she turned back to drinking.

Countless external circumstances can spark the urge to drink — a romantic breakup, job loss, new employment, a birth, a wedding, or any life transition. But it's not the events that lead to relapse; instead, it's our internal resistance to feeling our emotions about these events.

After 20 years sober, my mother's passing triggered a profound urge to drink. The taste of my old solace was almost palpable. But this wasn't just about loss — it was the realization that a meaningful mother-child relationship would never be. Mourning my mother's physical absence was one thing, but grieving the lack of a deeper emotional connection was heart-wrenching.

Some professionals contend that "relapse is part of recovery." While it's true that relapse may occur along the path to recovery, it's also true that it's not a mandatory checkpoint. The stark reality for those grappling with severe substance abuse issues is that a relapse might mean not making it back to sobriety at all. The addict's mind can be cunning, luring us into a false sense of security, whispering that everything will be alright. This is the difficult allure of addiction's psychological grip.

The paramount step is to embark on a journey of self-discovery. Take incremental steps toward introspection rather than external distraction. Embrace acceptance — of your identity, actions, and trajectory — as it is fundamental to enduring sobriety. Engage with the remarkable individual you are at this moment. Getting to know — and appreciate — the authentic you is vital to a fulfilling and sober life!

Developing a relapse prevention plan

A comprehensive relapse prevention plan is your roadmap to sustained sobriety. This personalized plan should encompass various coping mechanisms suited to different situations. From stress reduction techniques such as meditation and moderate exercise to building a robust support network, these strategies ensure you can handle temptations and difficult moments.

Reflect on daily practices that nurture your mental and physical well-being in constructing your plan. A balanced diet, sufficient rest, and regular physical activity are not optional luxuries but fundamental necessities. Incorporating these habits fosters a balance, equipping you to counter the unpredictable waves of recovery with grace and composure.

Navigating your narrative: A relapse prevention plan

Your unique story, with its trials, triumphs, and lessons, must be documented. Crafting a relapse prevention plan is key to strengthening your resolve and anticipating the road ahead. This exercise will help you become the author of your recovery, know your character, understand your plot twists, and prepare for the next chapters. This is your invitation to embark on a reflective and proactive quest to *own your story* and safeguard your sobriety.

>> **Character study — introspective inventory:** Set aside some quiet time. With a notebook or digital device, delve into an introspective inventory of your emotions, behaviors, and thoughts that have previously led to a relapse or might lead to one in the future.

>> **Plot points — recognizing triggers:** Identify your personal triggers (people, places, situations, emotions) and note them down. Be as specific as you can — each detail helps you recognize the early signs of a potential relapse.

>> **Story arc — developing coping strategies:** For each spark (trigger), write down a corresponding coping strategy or a positive action you can take. These can range from calling a

supportive friend to practicing mindfulness or engaging in a hobby. The sky's the limit; it's your strategy.

>> **Setting the scene — creating a supportive environment:** Reflect on your immediate environment and its *influence* on your recovery. Write down the changes you can make to ensure they support your sobriety. This could include removing alcohol from your home or setting up a corner for meditation.

>> **Dialogue — effective communication:** Practice "I" statements that you can use in stressful situations to express your feelings without blame. For example, "I feel overwhelmed when. . . and I need. . ."

>> **Climax — embracing high-risk situations:** Think about how you've handled high-risk situations in the past and how you wish to handle them moving forward. Make a plan for future scenarios, deciding in advance what your sober response will be.

>> **Denouement — post-relapse analysis:** In case of a relapse, use this section to analyze what happened. What led to it? What could you do differently? This is not about self-blame but about learning and preparing for the future.

>> **Epilogue — celebrating milestones:** Acknowledge and celebrate your sobriety milestones, no matter how small. Reward yourself with non-substance-related activities that bring you joy.

>> **Appendices — resources and support:** Compile a list of resources, hotlines, support groups, and contacts you can turn to in need.

>> **Continuous editing — revisiting your plan:** Make it a habit to revisit and revise your relapse prevention plan regularly. As you grow in your recovery, your needs may change, and your plan should evolve, too.

Incorporate this exercise into your recovery toolkit and revisit it often. With each review and revision, you reinforce your commitment to sobriety and ensure that your story — one of resilience and personal growth — will have a continuing journey toward a fulfilling, substance-free life.

Complacency in late recovery and the risk of relapse

WARNING

As you embrace the journey of long-term recovery, it's important to address a subtle yet perilous pitfall that can arise — complacency. Complacency in late recovery is often overlooked because the immediate threat of relapse feels distant. However, this false sense of security can lead to a lapse in the diligent practices that have supported your sobriety.

Statistics on relapse rates vary, but research has consistently shown that the risk remains significant even after years of abstinence. According to some studies, individuals in recovery can face relapse rates of about 40–60 percent, which are similar to rates of relapse for other chronic illnesses such as diabetes or hypertension. These figures highlight the importance of vigilance and active engagement in recovery efforts.

Complacency may manifest in several ways:

>> **Reduction in self-care:** Neglecting personal hygiene, nutrition, exercise, or sleep regimens can cause a gradual return to old, maladaptive habits.

>> **Avoidance of self-reflection:** Steering clear of introspection or therapy sessions may indicate resistance to confronting the necessary questions for growth and healing.

>> **Stagnation in personal growth:** Not setting new goals or pursuing challenges can lead to a comfortable but dangerous plateau, potentially opening doors to old behaviors.

>> **Ignoring boundaries:** Loosening or crossing previously set boundaries with certain people or situations put in place to protect your sobriety can lead to relapse.

>> **Isolation from support systems:** Drifting away from support groups, mentors, or friends who have been integral to your recovery can remove essential safeguards.

REMEMBER

The path of recovery is not a destination but a continuous journey. Treat each day as an opportunity for growth, learning, and connection. The moment you feel secure might be the moment to double down on the strategies that have helped you thus far.

Always be mindful that complacency can be the silent challenge of long-term recovery, and actively counteract it by revisiting your goals, engaging with your support network, and maintaining the practices contributing to your sobriety and well-being.

Embracing resilience and personal growth after relapse

Instead of seeing the period following a relapse as a defeat, consider it a rich soil in which resilience and personal growth can flourish. It's a time that beckons for introspection, a time to acknowledge the strengths you possess, even amidst setbacks, and consciously implement necessary changes. Nurturing resilience stems from recognizing that setbacks are merely detours on the journey of recovery, each one providing valuable lessons and directions for growth.

Adopting a growth-oriented mindset is instrumental as it fosters a perspective where every experience, relapses included, is considered an integral part of learning. This mindset lets you identify what went amiss and what can be done differently. It prompts a reexamination of your life's patterns and choices, urging you to realign them with your recovery objectives.

To truly flourish post-relapse, welcoming change and actively promoting resilience is essential. This proactive stance is characterized by a commitment to adopt healthier habits, continue self-reflection, and seek support when needed. Such resilience is not inherent — it is cultivated through persistent effort and an unwavering belief in your ability to overcome challenges.

As you advance on your journey, every step taken in the name of resilience fortifies your determination to return to the path of sobriety and push beyond it, reaching new heights of personal development. Therefore, the post-relapse phase is not just about regaining lost ground; it's an opportunity to deepen your connection with yourself, enhance your understanding of your triggers and responses, and solidify your coping strategies.

By embracing the dynamism of change and nurturing resilience, you position yourself not merely to bounce back from a relapse but to bounce forward, emerging stronger and more self-assured. Through this process, you constantly evolve, becoming the most authentic and empowered version of yourself — sober, resilient, and self-aware.

REMEMBER

A relapse, while challenging, is not the end of your story — it's a powerful catalyst for transformation. Let it be the moment you recommit to your growth, harness your inner strength, and stride forward with resilience. Your journey in recovery is one of perpetual learning and personal evolution, with every setback serving as a stepping stone to a more enlightened self.

Chapter **11**

Healing Together: The Path to Rebuilding Trust and Strengthening Family Ties

Walking the path of sobriety is not something you do alone; your family and friends are there to support you, bringing their experiences and emotions to the collective effort. The journey can be challenging and complex, yet persistence leads to rebuilding trust and open conversation. Your efforts in recovery are about more than overcoming addiction; they're also about restoring and rebuilding relationships that may have been damaged. This is a chance to improve family bonds and support your dedication to a life without substances.

In this chapter, we'll explore the dynamics of trust and communication within your family, taking a close look at the ways addiction can affect these aspects of relationships. You'll gain valuable insights and strategies to support you and your loved ones rebuild trust and enhance communication. The aim is not just to avoid past mistakes but to actively learn better ways to interact, encourage openness, and put aside pride. This process shows your dedication to those who support you — that together, you will work on healing for mutual growth. You'll tackle the challenges of trust issues and the importance of setting boundaries as you explore a thorough approach to repair and strengthen your family connections during sobriety.

Rebuilding Trust and Communication

Trust is the foundation of the family, and good communication is critical to rebuilding that trust after it has been weakened by addiction. To heal together as a family, fostering conversation rooted in honesty and empathy is essential. It begins with an effort from all members to prioritize recovery and actively participate in the recovery journey, addressing habits and behaviors that may perpetuate a dry-drunk state wherein someone is abstaining from alcohol but not engaging in recovery. Recovery is a state of being and an active lifestyle choice.

Rebuilding trust requires honestly recognizing past behaviors and the hurt they caused. It's about owning your story, faults and all, and providing a safe space for each family member to communicate without fear of judgment. When trust begins to be re-established, relationships within the family can start to heal, growing stronger and more resilient than before. Encouraging openness and honesty, without excuses or defensiveness, paves the way for a nurturing environment.

REMEMBER

While it's important to avoid past triggers, it can also be helpful for family members to explore ways to communicate effectively. Active listening is a key technique — giving full attention without interrupting, making excuses, or letting emotions steer the conversation toward blame. Using "I" statements rather than accusations, maintaining eye contact to show engagement, pausing before responding to ensure thoughtful interaction, and even writing out important messages to prevent misunderstandings can be beneficial strategies. These approaches may contribute to a healthy recovery rooted in mutual trust and understanding.

Addressing trust issues within the family

Addressing trust issues within the family may feel daunting, but it's a crucial step toward healing. Trust, once damaged by the effects of addiction, leaves behind a trail of doubt and hurt. Rebuilding requires a deep dive into the underlying issues undermining the family structure, such as unaddressed emotions and offensive behavior. This self-reflection is not for the faint of heart. Still, it is necessary for those serious about recovery and re-establishing a sense of security within the family.

Creating an environment of trust means allowing family members to be vulnerable — sharing their struggles and their wins. Recognizing and addressing personal faults openly takes courage but is the path to an honest and authentic relationship with those closest to you. It's about creating a safe space where people can voice their feelings without fear of being used as weapons in future arguments.

As difficult as these conversations may be, they are pivotal for strengthening family ties. Ensuring each family member feels heard and understood without judgment instills a sense of belonging and togetherness. When efforts are made to understand each other's emotional responses, the likelihood of resolving conflicts with compassion increases tremendously, steering the family unit toward a more cohesive and trusting dynamic.

Effective communication strategies in recovery

Recovery is more than abstinence; it's about engaging in a transformative process that affects every aspect of one's life, including communication with family. Active participation in recovery involves embracing strategies that elevate communication beyond the superficial. This means integrating the practice of using "I" statements, thereby fostering an environment where thoughts and feelings can be expressed without casting blame. "I feel" rather than "You make me feel" shifts the dialogue from accusation to personal experience, opening the door to empathy and understanding.

Drawing from the rich insight we've uncovered, let's craft a simple exercise designed to reinforce effective communication strategies in recovery. Imagine this as a mini-workshop activity to slide into the chapter you're writing, bringing to life the concepts of using "I" statements and being fully present.

Communication reflection

Now, let's practice being present during conversations and becoming more aware of how we express our thoughts and feelings. You'll need a notebook and pen (or any digital device).

Follow these instructions:

1. **Find your space:** Look for a quiet spot where you can sit undisturbed. This will be your stage for introspection and practice.

2. **Take a reflective pause:** Close your eyes and take three deep breaths. With each inhalation, imagine pulling in clarity; release any tension or preconceived notions about communication with each exhalation.

3. **Practice self-dialogue:** Think of a recent conversation that didn't go as well as you'd hoped, maybe one that left you feeling misunderstood or unheard.

- Write down what you said using "you" statements, for instance, "You didn't take my feelings into account."

- Now, rewrite the statement using "I" language, such as, "I felt hurt because I didn't feel considered in the discussion."

- Reflect on the difference between the two statements. How do the "I" statements change the tone and impact of the message?

4. **Practice being present:** Recall the same conversation but focus on how present you were. Were you fully engaged, or was your mind elsewhere?

   Write down one action you could take next time to be more present. It might be as simple as turning off your phone or reminding yourself to maintain eye contact.

5. **Role-play in your mind:** Imagine the conversation happening again, this time using the "I" statements and the action you identified to be more present.

   Visualize the outcome. How does your conversation partner react to the changes in your approach?

6. **Commit to action:** Pledge to apply these strategies in your next conversation. It may feel a bit awkward initially, but remember, practice is the path to proficiency.

7. **Debrief:** After implementing these strategies in a real conversation, take a moment to journal about the experience. Did the strategies improve the communication? Did you feel more connected and understood?

It's not just about changing words; it's about shifting perspective. By owning your feelings and experiences, you invite dialogue instead of defensiveness. Being present can be a superpower in communication — it shows the other person they have your full attention, often leading to a more meaningful exchange.

By putting these strategies into practice, you're honing your communication skills and cultivating a nurturing environment that supports recovery and strengthens relationships. Now, who knew a simple swap from "you" to "I" and a moment of mindfulness could do so much? Go ahead, give it a shot, and watch your conversations transform!

REMEMBER

Being fully present is essential in communication. It's easy to be swept away by daily life's constant distractions or preoccupied with personal thoughts and worries. However, making an effort to engage fully in the moment, making eye contact, and really hearing what the other person is saying can transform a simple conversation into a powerful tool for healing. It's about pausing before speaking, allowing for the opportunity to digest what's been heard and respond with mindfulness.

In addition to interpersonal communication, family therapy and counseling play a significant role in recovery. These professional avenues provide education and support, helping family members understand the complexities of addiction as a family disease. By participating in therapy, families can learn customized strategies to rebuild and strengthen their unique dynamic, enabling them to become a robust support system for each other as they navigate the path of recovery.

Family therapy and counseling

Understanding that recovery from addiction cannot occur in isolation but thrives through collaborative effort is key. Therefore, family therapy and counseling are crucial for healing. As you engage in family counseling, there's an acknowledgment that addiction affects each member of the family differently. In the safe environment created by therapists, you can explore the complex relationship between personal traumas, relationship dynamics, and addictive behaviors. Here, your family will learn to deconstruct the stigmas attached to addiction, view it through the lens of empathy, and collectively adopt approaches to prevent relapse and nurture recovery.

In addition, workshops and group therapy activities extend beyond mere dialogue, prompting experiential learning about addiction and its impact. Your family can participate in role-playing exercises, education modules, and support group discussions. These experiences help you see addiction as a chronic, relapsing condition that requires strong, informed family support. Through therapy and counseling, you learn how everyone's recovery is connected to the family's overall health, helping you heal together and build a supportive, lasting environment.

Education and Support for Family Members

Recognizing addiction as a struggle that affects the whole family, not just the individual, is the first step in creating a supportive environment. Addiction affects familial bonds, leaving no relationship untouched. By acknowledging this common struggle, you pave the way for a united effort against the widespread impact of addiction. Learning about addiction with your family is key to building empathy and supporting long-term recovery.

The family must understand that as you navigate the journey of recovery, your struggles with addiction are not a matter of willpower or moral failing but rather a chronic disease that requires comprehensive treatment and ongoing management. Education paves the way to understanding the difference between enabling behaviors and supportive ones, enhancing the quality of the help they offer. Just as the person in recovery requires guidance and assistance, you and your family need resources to recognize the signs of relapse, learn strategies for effective communication, and understand the importance of setting healthy boundaries.

FROM SOBRIETY TO FAMILY RENEWAL WITH AMY

My journey to sobriety was deeply personal, unfolding within the walls of our family home under the watchful eyes of my loved ones. It began with a yearning to heal and reclaim my sense of wholeness, yet I soon realized that recovery was more intricate than I had anticipated. My family witnessed the complicated steps like attending meetings and juggling childcare and the heartening moments when I began to transform, demonstrating my resilience and resolve.

When it came to discussing my past and ongoing sobriety with my children, I walked slowly with care, aiming to educate them without instilling fear. My story wasn't just mine; it also served as a lesson and hope for my family. My transformation had a profound effect, particularly on my youngest son, who, at a pivotal point in his life journey, was moved to write an essay about the resilience and change he saw in me.

My vigilant eyes watched for signs of addiction's reach toward my children, but my experiences granted me a unique credibility that extended beyond the realm of typical parental guidance. I could empathize and forge genuine connections with my family on these matters.

(continued)

(continued)

As I progressed, it became necessary to confront the repercussions of my past behaviors. Yet, through living with greater openness and integrity, I began to mend my ties with my family, especially with my eldest daughter. Our heartfelt conversations drew us closer, and she honored my sobriety date with a tattoo, symbolizing a fresh beginning for us all.

My sobriety journey entailed more than abstaining from alcohol — it transformed me and resonated with everyone around me. I showed my family that while I didn't possess all the answers, I had acquired the tools to navigate life's ebbs and flows. My narrative is more than a tale of overcoming addiction; it illustrates how personal trials can illuminate a path for others, fostering a space of vulnerability and connection and fortifying the bonds within our family.

REMEMBER

Providing a safe space for open dialogue is another crucial element in rebuilding trust and strengthening connections. Talking openly about feelings, fears, and expectations helps everyone address the challenges that addiction presents.

Lastly, involvement in support groups can offer you and your family invaluable companionship and learning opportunities from others who are on similar paths. In these groups, you can collectively explore the principles of recovery, share successes and setbacks, and gain new perspectives. Such collective experiences promote the notion that addiction recovery is a communal journey, not to be taken on by any single family member alone. The community spirit builds resilience and encourages you to rely on collective wisdom to heal together.

Understanding addiction as a family disease

Addiction not only affects the individual struggling with the substance but also casts a shadow over the entire family unit. It's as if a once peaceful household finds itself amid an emotional storm, where every family member's well-being is compromised. If your loved one is struggling with addiction, it's important to understand that you are not just an observer but part of a system that addiction has disrupted. Understanding this is a key first step to healing, as it changes recovery from a lone struggle to a collective effort of renewal and growth.

Through this shared perspective, you and your family can begin to unite against the disruptive force of addiction. Seeing addiction as a family disease means acknowledging that everyone plays a role in the recovery process. It involves setting aside blame and recognizing that the behaviors and patterns established within the family may have unknowingly contributed to or been affected by the addiction. Doing so creates an environment where each family member feels seen, heard, and empowered to contribute to the collective healing. Establishing open lines of communication and setting healthy boundaries become not just strategies but acts of love and commitment to each other's well-being.

REMEMBER

Embracing the concept of addiction as a family disease also necessitates a journey toward education and understanding. As you and your family become more informed about the nature of addiction, it becomes clearer that it's a chronic illness requiring ongoing attention and compassion. With knowledge, your family can turn the challenges of addiction into a force for growth and resilience.

Providing resources and information for families

Equipping you and your family with the requisite knowledge to navigate recovery is paramount to the journey ahead. Much like venturing into the wilderness armed with a reliable map and compass, educating yourselves about the nuances of addiction, recovery, and mental illness lays the groundwork for a successful expedition toward healing. By using resources on addiction, communication, and conflict resolution, you can turn your home from a battleground into a place of comfort. Here are some ideas of resources you can look into:

>> **Books and articles on addiction and recovery:** Curate a list of key readings that offer insights into the biological, psychological, and social aspects of addiction, along with personal stories of recovery and resilience.

>> **Online courses and webinars:** Recommend online learning opportunities that focus on understanding addiction, improving communication skills, and effective strategies for conflict resolution.

>> **Support groups and workshops:** List both local and online support groups and workshops for families affected by addiction, such as Al-Anon, Nar-Anon, or family therapy workshops.

>> **Toolkits for effective communication:** Provide guides or toolkits that teach families how to communicate effectively, including how to listen actively, speak openly, and handle sensitive topics.

>> **Professional counseling and therapy services:** Offer information on finding and choosing therapists specializing in addiction and family dynamics, including directories or networks for licensed professionals.

REMEMBER

Your role in recovery is active, not passive. Actively gathering and understanding resources helps you navigate the recovery landscape, including the dry-drunk and emotional versus physical sobriety concepts. A dry drunk is someone who has stopped drinking alcohol but still acts in ways that were common during their drinking days, such as being angry or impulsive.

Engaging with educational materials, individually or in seminars, builds a shared understanding and vocabulary, facilitating a platform for open expression of feelings without fear of judgment. Effective communication through active listening, using "I" statements, and being present strengthens family trust, promoting open dialogue. Rebuilding trust also involves creating a safe space where everyone feels heard, owning up to past mistakes, and committing to personal growth. Using resources strategically is crucial for managing sensitive issues constructively. Additionally, support groups expand your support network, offering broader perspectives and community engagement, enhancing the recovery journey.

Family support groups and networks

Support groups and networks provide essential reinforcement for you and your family as you confront the challenges presented by long-term recovery from addiction. Within these communities, you find a safe space for exchanging stories, revealing struggles, and acquiring knowledge from others navigating recovery. Participation in support groups grants you a feeling of community and access to a wealth of shared understanding, which can be invaluable during difficult periods and when you need additional strength to maintain your sobriety.

In the confusion of addiction, it's easy to feel alone and powerless. However, family support groups act as a guiding light, leading you to a community where understanding and sympathy are abundant. Within these groups, you'll find like-minded people who have navigated addiction themselves. They know the pain of betrayal and the weight of disappointment. In these gatherings, every share and every nod signifies you're not alone, offering a compassionate space where your struggles are met with empathy, not judgment.

As you engage with these networks, you discover the strength of healing together. The shared stories are about struggle, victory, and resilience. The collective insight and encouragement of the group nourish your journey of recovery. These encounters foster open communication and an understanding of addiction not just as your battle but as a family disease that impacts everyone involved. By acknowledging this, families begin to reconstruct trust and piece together the shattered pieces of their bonds.

TIP

Engaging with these groups gives you tools and strategies that are hard to find when struggling alone. You discover how to set boundaries, communicate effectively using "I" language, and positively recognize and address offensive behaviors. Support groups can deepen your understanding and improve family dynamics, acting as stepping stones for your family's recovery and renewal.

Establishing Healthy Family Dynamics

In recognizing the importance of family support, you can explore a multifaceted approach to rebuild trust and strengthen family ties after addiction and recovery.

Setting boundaries to create a supportive environment and encouraging open, honest dialogue are crucial to repairing broken family ties. You will explore communication practices that build trust and collaboration, such as active listening and avoiding dry-drunk behaviors that can block progress.

REMEMBER

This journey is not without challenges; confronting our own faults and extending effort and vulnerability is essential for making "living amends." By showcasing the significance of consistent behavior, we provide insight into how every action can contribute to a stronger, more resilient family dynamic. Families can heal together with dedication, patience, and the right set of tools.

Setting boundaries for a supportive environment

In the journey toward healing, one of the first steps is to create a supportive environment that fosters recovery. This involves the implementation of transparent and firm boundaries, which can be a dynamic process of understanding and negotiation within the family. Trust starts to grow within these boundaries by ensuring the needs of the person seeking sobriety and other family members are recognized and respected. Boundaries may address personal space, accountability, acceptable behaviors, and details such as ensuring quiet times for reflection and recovery work.

These boundaries go beyond setting rules; they are declarations of a family's commitment to the well-being of all its members. Establishing these boundaries should involve all family members, including defining consequences for when they are crossed. Adjusting to these new dynamics can feel rigid at first, but with time, the family can move toward a sense of normalcy and respect for each recovery journey. As challenging as it may be, this structure is often necessary to protect the delicate balance of trust and foster a space where healing can flourish.

REMEMBER

One must not confuse boundaries with walls. The goal is not to isolate or constrain but to create a nurturing space where the temptation of old habits can be kept at bay, enabling behaviors to be prevented and recovery to take priority. It's a delicate balance that requires commitment and open communication. The more honest families are with each other in this process, the more they can create an atmosphere conducive to everyone's growth and healing.

Encouraging openness and honesty in the family

For families on the path of healing, openness and honesty are as important as setting boundaries. These qualities foster deep understanding and empathy, strengthening family bonds. True healing demands transparency, allowing members to freely share their feelings and concerns without fear of judgment. This involves breaking down past defensive behaviors and reflective tendencies that were once coping mechanisms. Active listening is essential, especially when emotions and misunderstandings are likely. Families can build a new level of trust by striving to understand each other before being understood and expressing emotions through various means like writing.

REMEMBER

Building this trust through honesty and openness is a gradual process. It requires individuals to acknowledge their past actions, communicate effectively, and listen without defensiveness. As family dynamics improve, the journey of healing together shifts from a mere goal to a daily practice. This ongoing effort enriches every interaction, conversation, and decision, steering the family toward a future of collective well-being and stability.

Chapter **12**

Building a Career and Gaining Employment

I n the dynamic landscape of your career, your sobriety is like a lighthouse, shining a steady light that helps you navigate through the fog of uncertainty toward a career path that is fulfilling and true to your values. As you craft your sober-friendly career plan, remember you are the captain of your professional journey. Your sobriety doesn't limit your potential; it enriches it, providing the clear vision necessary to make choices that align with your career aspirations and your commitment to a healthier way of living. Just as a compass points north, let your values and goals steer your career decisions toward workplaces that respect and support your decision to live alcohol-free.

In this chapter, you're invited to an expedition to map out a career that sustains you financially and supports your sober lifestyle. We'll explore strategies for finding and thriving in environments that respect your boundaries and celebrate your strengths. You'll learn how to communicate your needs effectively, ensuring you don't have to navigate the professional waters alone.

Crafting a Sober-Friendly Career Plan

Embarking on a formidable path of career building while steadily maintaining your sobriety can be likened to navigating a river's unpredictable currents — challenging but not impossible. Your career plan should serve as a compass, guiding you toward professional goals that resonate deeply with your values and support your sober lifestyle. The initial step is consciously avoiding workplaces and not supporting your sobriety journey. Seek out and take advantage of non-alcoholic alternatives at work events, and don't shy away from communicating your needs to the HR department. Remember, your sobriety doesn't diminish your capabilities; instead, it can offer a newfound clarity and focus to channel into your professional endeavors.

As you move ahead, the importance of open and honest communication about your sobriety cannot be overstated. This forthrightness can pave the way for a supportive work culture and free you from the stress of concealing a significant part of your life. Use workplace support systems to your advantage — dialogue with HR and your managers to create a safety net that empowers you. Such environments respect your journey and leverage your unique strengths, which, in turn, can drive your career development and advancement. Setting clear, achievable goals and committing to continuous learning can lead to substantial professional growth and maybe even a role you had never envisioned for yourself.

As you continue to build a sober career path and gain fulfilling employment, crafting a sober-friendly career plan supporting your recovery journey is essential. The following questions are designed to help you align your career aspirations with your commitment to sobriety. Take time to reflect on each question; your responses will serve as a foundation for a fulfilling and supportive professional path.

Crafting a sober-friendly career plan questionnaire

There are no right or wrong answers, only what feels true to your journey and goals.

» **Assessing your current state:** At this point in your recovery, how do you feel about re-entering the workforce or pursuing a new career trajectory?

» **Understanding sobriety compatibility:** What are the most critical aspects of a job that would support and not jeopardize your sobriety?

» **Identifying potential sparks (triggers):** Are there specific work environments, industries, or job roles that might challenge your sobriety?

» **Creating a work-life balance:** How do you plan to balance work demands with your recovery efforts to maintain a healthy lifestyle?

» **Identifying skill sets and interests:** What are your essential skills and interests, and how can they be applied to a career conducive to your sobriety?

» **Setting career aspirations:** Where do you see yourself professionally in one, five, and ten years?

» **Leveraging networking and support:** How can you leverage your support network in your career development? Do you need guidance on networking sober?

» **Engaging in professional development:** What additional training or education might you need to achieve your career goals while prioritizing your sobriety?

» **Preventing relapse:** How will your career plan include strategies to prevent relapse, such as stress management and self-care?

» **Setting your disclosure plan:** What's your approach to disclosing (or not disclosing) your recovery to potential employers?

» **Identifying non-negotiables:** What elements must be present in your work environment to ensure they align with your recovery values?

>> **Have a long-term vision:** How does your career plan contribute to the person you wish to become in long-term sobriety?

>> **Align your career with recovery:** Explore the intersection of what you love, what you are good at, and what the world needs through the Ikigai framework to discover a career that energizes and fulfills you. If you haven't worked with a career coach, now may be a time to consider enlisting one to fine-tune your professional growth and ensure your job trajectory complements your sober lifestyle. Use this time of personal reinvention to seek out roles that resonate with your values and contribute to a meaningful, satisfying work life.

TIP

It's imperative to tailor your career pursuits based on *intrinsic* interests rather than extrinsic rewards to ensure resilient alignment with your recovery. Take time for self-reflection; identify careers that energize you and align with your mission. The Ikigai exercise from Chapter 9 is an exceptional tool that can help elucidate your passions, strengths, and values, bridging them with the professional world. This personal alignment might even prompt a career transition that aligns better with your sober life — a brave step fostered through self-teaching and thoughtful class selection. Don't discount the value of a career coach who can provide expert guidance on developing your skills and strategically ask for raises or promotions. Your journey in recovery is a potent time to explore new interests, reinvent yourself, and ultimately, construct a career that doesn't just make a living but enriches your life.

Identifying career interests and passions

Before anything else, take a moment to assess your skills, interests, and passions. This self-reflection, made more accessible through exercises such as Ikigai, can reveal much about the direction in which your career might most naturally flourish. Remember, now is the time to explore new interests that recovery has afforded you the space to uncover. Look for career possibilities that resonate with you and inherently avoid environments with potential triggers, like alcohol. This initial step is about creating a solid foundation for a future where you feel vibrant and alive at work and in your sobriety.

Delving into your interests and passions is akin to unlocking a map to your professional well-being. Reflect on what activities make you lose track of time, the topics you're eager to read about, or the kinds of conversations that energize you. Your career should not just be a job but a journey that *aligns* with your core values and brings you fulfillment. As you consider various paths, consider how your work can contribute to your sobriety journey, reinforcing your commitment to a healthier life.

REMEMBER

Before embarking on your career journey, invest time in self-reflection and understanding what brings you joy and purpose. An exercise like Ikigai can illuminate your path, guiding you toward a profession that aligns with your recovery, fulfills you, and keeps you engaged. Your career should be an extension of your passion and values, complementing your commitment to sobriety and enhancing your well-being.

Mapping out your career trajectory in the context of recovery requires careful consideration. You might discover that you're naturally drawn to roles emphasizing support and community — positions where you can use your experiences to uplift others. Or perhaps you find motivation in creative outlets that demand innovation and original thought. Engage in networking, seek feedback from trusted peers or a career coach, and evaluate how your strengths can serve you professionally. This feedback loop is crucial as it often highlights skills you undervalue or haven't fully realized.

As you identify your passions and interests, consider the practical side of your career planning. While it's important to pursue what you love, ensure that your chosen path includes the potential for growth, stability, and the chance to learn and develop new skills continuously. Building a career while sober is not just about avoiding triggers; it's about creating a rewarding and sustainable life. Integrating your passions with a viable career option will enhance your professional journey and bolster your sobriety with a meaningful and inspiring day-to-day existence.

TIP

While career planning in recovery, leverage your unique experiences and strengths in a profession promoting personal growth and community support, enhancing your career and recovery journey. Embrace feedback, network actively, and consult with a career coach to uncover hidden talents and align your career with your passions. Balance your aspirations with practical considerations, seeking roles that offer stability and opportunities for lifelong learning, thereby crafting a sustainable career that nourishes your sobriety.

Aligning career goals with sobriety

When it comes to aligning your career goals with your sobriety, it's essential to acknowledge how integral your journey to recovery is to your professional success. Your sobriety shapes more than just your personal life; it impacts every decision, including your career path. Start by evaluating your professional environment and the roles you undertake. Ask yourself whether these settings support or threaten your sobriety. If you're frequently exposed to environments with alcohol, it might be time to seek a career shift — one that respects and enhances your commitment to a sober lifestyle. This also offers the chance to explore roles that are not only safe but also fulfilling by harnessing your strengths.

Equipping your workplace with the knowledge of your sobriety can seem daunting, but it paves the way for mutual understanding and support. Exercise openness by communicating with your HR department about your needs for non-alcoholic options at events. This dialogue often leads to broader discussions about inclusive practices that benefit everyone. Embrace the clarity and dedication that sobriety brings to your work ethic; it could lead to more meaningful connections with colleagues and career advancement opportunities that align with your values.

While rooted in your victory, your sobriety can be a lever for professional growth. In your journey, make sure to leverage the perspectives of trusted peers and mentors to gain insights into how your strengths — perhaps sharpened by the challenges you've overcome — can be applied to your career ambitions. This exercise reinforces your commitment to sobriety and highlights the unique attributes you bring to the table. Choosing a career that resonates with your passion and supports your sober lifestyle sets you up for rewarding and sustainable success.

TIP

Align your career goals with sobriety. Assess your work environment and roles for their compatibility with your sobriety, and consider a shift if necessary to protect your recovery. Engage with your workplace to foster an understanding of your needs, advocating for inclusive practices that support your sober lifestyle. Utilize your sobriety as a foundation for professional growth, allowing the strengths and insights gained from your journey to inform your career choices and fuel a fulfilling and sustainable path forward.

Building a career plan with recovery in mind

When it's time to put pen to paper or fingers to keyboard, remember that recovery grants you challenges and opportunities. Your journey to sobriety is a powerful testament to your resilience and strength, invaluable qualities in the workforce. As you consider your career trajectory, set tangible goals for development and advancement that account for continuous learning and skill development. Whether you're looking to climb the corporate ladder or carve out a new professional path, embrace your experience in recovery as the compass that steers you toward choices aligned with your well-being and values.

Keep in mind that pursuing a career while maintaining sobriety can require strategic avoidance of certain environments. Armed with a clear understanding of what settings to circumvent and when to utilize a sober companion, you can craft a career that's both fulfilling and safe. Engaging your workplace's support systems is essential, and communicating transparently with HR and managers to ensure accommodations that respect your needs is essential. As you advocate for a sober-friendly work culture, you might find that initiatives such as including non-alcoholic options at events can be both personally beneficial and widely appreciated by colleagues.

REMEMBER

A career pivot or advancement in the context of recovery is possible and can be a profound chapter of your life. Recovery time allows for self-reflection and the chance to explore new interests and passions, which can translate into exciting career opportunities. Utilize resources such as career coaching, skills assessments, and educational opportunities to build and refine the toolkit you need for the job market. Viewing your ambitions through the lens of recovery ensures a plan that not only charts a course for professional success but also safeguards your sobriety — ultimately leading to sustainable personal growth and fulfillment.

Your ambitions are achievable with the right support and a plan that's mindful of your sobriety. By integrating your recovery journey into your career planning, you are setting the stage for a professional life that is not only successful but also enriching and true to your identity. This integration ensures a holistic approach, where you don't have to choose between career growth and your personal needs, but rather, you create a roadmap to achieve both professional success and personal well-being.

Career development at each stage of sobriety

Aligning your career goals with your sobriety is an evolving process that continues to unfold as you grow in your recovery. Your aspirations will likely shift as you reach different milestones, reshaping your outlook and objectives.

» **One-year mark — discovery and foundation building:** During your first year, your primary focus is likely on discovering who you are without the influence of alcohol or substances. This is a time of rebuilding and laying down a new foundation for your career. You may find exploring various interests and taking stock of your strengths and skills beneficial. Engaging in a career that supports your recovery environment is crucial, as is avoiding potential triggers.

» **Five-year mark — growth and expansion:** By the five-year milestone, you've likely solidified your new identity in sobriety and started to see growth in your professional life. This phase often brings an increasing desire for career advancement or even a change in direction that better aligns with your core values. It's an optimal time to reassess your goals and aspirations, ensuring they harmonize with your sober lifestyle.

>> **Ten-year mark — mastery and purpose:** You might seek deeper meaning and purpose in your career a decade into recovery. It's common to strive for mastery in your field or to leverage your experiences to make a broader impact, such as mentoring others or engaging in advocacy. Your professional goals might be about advancement, legacy, and contribution.

>> **Beyond ten years — legacy and sustained success:** As you move beyond ten years of sobriety, you're likely looking at the bigger picture of your career trajectory. This could involve cementing your legacy within your profession and ensuring that your work continues to align with the principles supporting your recovery. Sustained success in your career also means continued investment in your personal development and wellness, which remains a cornerstone of long-term sobriety.

At each stage, your aspirations act as a compass, guiding your decisions to ensure that your career moves in tandem with your sobriety journey. Regular self-reflection and consultation with trusted mentors can help you navigate these evolving goals, always prioritizing your recovery.

As you progress through your journey in recovery, it is important to remain vigilant against complacency, a common challenge that can emerge at any stage. Complacency often creeps in quietly, masquerading as confidence or a sense of security in one's sobriety. However, this false sense of security can lead to a relaxation of recovery efforts and, potentially, to relapse.

As discussed in earlier chapters, particularly when exploring the neuroscience of addiction and the importance of continuous self-reflection and growth (refer to chapters 4 and 15), your brain has undergone significant changes during addiction, and it continues to heal and adapt during recovery. Complacency can hinder this ongoing process by stalling your commitment to the practices that support your sobriety, such as mindfulness, regular attendance at support group meetings, or engaging in healthy lifestyle choices.

In the first year of recovery, focus on establishing a strong foundation that includes understanding your triggers, building a solid support network, and developing healthy coping mechanisms. This groundwork is vital for sustaining long-term sobriety.

By the five-year mark, you should be actively working on personal growth, setting new goals, and possibly taking on new roles that align with your sober identity. This is the time to reassess your aspirations to ensure they still serve your sober lifestyle and to adjust them if necessary.

At the ten-year milestone, you've likely achieved a level of comfort and confidence in your recovery. This is a critical period to guard against complacency by seeking new challenges that promote personal development and prevent stagnation.

As you move beyond a decade of sobriety, consider your legacy and the long-term impact of your career choices on your recovery. Now is the time to mentor others, give back to the recovery community, and ensure the sustainability of your achievements.

REMEMBER

Recovery is a lifelong journey, and your aspirations will evolve along with it. Always prioritize your sobriety and refer to the chapters on developing coping mechanisms (chapters 2 and 14) and the neuroscience of addiction and continuous learning in recovery (chapters 5, 8, and 15) as guides to help you navigate each stage of this fulfilling journey.

Navigating the Job Search and Interviews Sober

As you embark on the job search, your sobriety is a beacon guiding your way to employment and a career that enhances your recovery lifestyle. Searching for a job is more than scanning listings — it's a deliberate process of aligning prospective roles with your sober narrative. Start by identifying companies that champion work-life balance and have a culture of inclusivity. When researching organizations, look beyond their success in the market and delve into their policies on substance-free work environments and employee support programs. These elements are not merely perks but foundations for a sustainable career that resonates with your values.

The interview stage offers unique challenges and opportunities for someone in recovery. It's a moment where authenticity and preparation merge, allowing you to portray your commitment to sobriety as a strength. When fielding questions about employment gaps or why you left your last position, frame your answers positively, highlighting the skills and insights you've gained from your recovery. Remember, you are not obligated to disclose your sobriety. However, if you choose to, do so confidently as part of your story — show how it has empowered you, leading to personal growth and professional reliability.

Moreover, don't underestimate the value of being selective. An integral part of the job hunt is recognizing which environments might jeopardize your recovery and steering clear of them, regardless of the allure of the role or the prestige of the company. Seek out mentors or career coaches who can help you craft a clear vision of your ideal career path — one that not only accepts but celebrates your journey toward sobriety. Use your network to uncover opportunities that match your lifestyle, and during interviews, inquire about the company's perspectives on health and wellness to ensure their principles align with your needs.

Navigating the job search while sober is not just about landing a job; it's a proactive stride toward a life that honors your commitment to recovery. With each step, you can build a career that's more than a paycheck — it's a testament to your resilience and dedication to a brighter future.

Effective job search strategies for individuals in recovery

Your journey through recovery has gifted you with a level of resilience and mental strength that many employers find admirable. While you're out there charting the course of your new career, remember that networking is your beacon. Regularly attending networking events is crucial for your contacts and the personal growth and confidence you'll build. However, if the faces in the crowd start to look too familiar, it might be time to cast your net in different waters. Don't hesitate to look for new networking groups or events to reinvigorate your job search. This helps you avoid feeling stuck and propels you forward, opening up newer, more diverse professional avenues that align with your renewed outlook on life.

Creating a work environment that is conducive to your sobriety is paramount. You've worked hard to reach this stage; your workplace should support that. When discussing options with potential employers, be upfront about your preference for non-alcoholic events and see if they're willing and able to collaborate with HR to create an inclusive and supportive office culture. Your openness about your sobriety can be liberating and can set the stage for a genuinely comfortable and productive work atmosphere that respects your lifestyle choices.

Professional growth doesn't halt during recovery; in fact, this period can be a springboard for career development. Setting clear, reachable goals will provide a roadmap to advancing in your career. Continually seeking to enhance your skill set is integral to your professional journey — investing in a career coach may be worthwhile. A coach can provide the external perspective and expertise needed to navigate the tricky waters of professional advancement. They can assist you with everything from fine-tuning your resume to preparing for interviews and negotiating the salary that reflects your worth. Remember, your value in the workplace is immense, and you owe it to yourself to be compensated fairly and competitively.

Addressing employment gaps and recovery in interviews

When discussing employment gaps in interviews, your approach should hinge on honesty and framing your recovery as a transformative journey. It's important to remember that every person has their own unique narrative, and your experience with recovery is a powerful testament to your strength and determination. Articulate the period away from the workforce as one of personal growth, highlighting that the time spent was essential for developing a greater sense of self-awareness and fortitude. This can resonate with employers who value personal development and human resilience.

As you prepare to talk about your employment gaps, consider the personal attributes you've honed during your recovery. Your journey has likely instilled in you an extraordinary level of discipline, a profound ability to focus on goals, and an admirable dedication to self-improvement. These are all qualities that are highly sought after in the professional world. When you craft your narrative, ensure you confidently convey these strengths. By doing so, you demonstrate that you didn't merely take a hiatus from work but underwent a period of strategic life better-ment that has prepared you to contribute meaningfully to the workplace.

Your recovery is a personal aspect of your life, and you have sole discretion over how much to share professionally. If you choose to disclose your sobriety, do so in a manner that underscores how it has positively impacted your professional abilities. Be selective with the details and focus on how your recovery has led to an improved work ethic, enhanced problem-solving skills, or a more profound commitment to your career.

REMEMBER

Shedding light on your journey is not a liability; it's an opportunity to illustrate your development into a more adaptive and insightful professional. Strategic disclosure can pave the way for a workplace environment that is more inclusive and supportive of diverse life experiences.

In every interview, your primary goal is to convince the employer that you are the best candidate. Address any employment gaps with poised assurance, presenting them as deliberate pauses that have equipped you with unique insights and capabilities that others may lack. Your recovery is not a detour but a deep drive within you that has now been channeled into professional and personal excellence. In framing your past challenges as pillars of your current strength, you exchange vulnerability for valor, crafting a compelling narrative that positions you as a candidate and an aspirant with invaluable lived experiences.

Disclosing sobriety in the workplace

Deciding whether to share your sobriety journey with your col-leagues is an act of personal bravery and authenticity. It's an individual decision that carries its weight for each person. When you disclose your sobriety at work, you open up a space for understanding and can set an exemplary standard of honesty and trust within your team. It also allows you to navigate work events with a straightforward narrative for why you decline alcohol and can help in aligning with others who support your choices or are on a similar path.

Communication with your HR department about your sobriety can play a key role in ensuring you receive appropriate support in the workplace. Expressing your needs for non-alcoholic alternatives at company events and meetings not only benefits you but can also influence inclusive event planning that respects everyone's lifestyle choices. Your experience in sobriety equips you with distinct insights and strengths that can enhance your professional relationships. By confidently sharing your status, you encourage a work culture that values diversity in personal journeys and builds deeper connections among coworkers.

Creating a dialogue around sobriety in the workplace does more than just inform — it educates and can dismantle stereotypes. Your decision to be open about your recovery is a powerful acknowledgment of your commitment to self-improvement. It is a testament to your dedication, resilience, and the proactive strides you've made in personal growth. Reflect carefully on your company's environment and the possible repercussions, knowing that your well-being and comfort should remain paramount as you share your truth. Ultimately, your courage in disclosing your sobriety at work can become a cornerstone of your professional identity, inspiring others and enhancing the collective understanding of recovery.

Thriving in the Workplace Sober

Your journey toward a fulfilling career in sobriety is about more than just staying away from alcohol; it's about creating an environment where your well-being is a priority. In the early stages of recovery, it can be challenging to navigate workplace situations where alcohol is present. However, with a well-thought-out approach, you can confidently assert your needs. Know that it's perfectly acceptable to avoid events or settings that might put your sobriety at risk, and if you choose to attend, having a sober companion by your side can be an immense support. As you grow more comfortable in your sobriety, you'll also find strength in the ability to socialize without feeling the need to drink, opening doors to new social and professional opportunities.

Building a sober-friendly career involves proactive communication and planning. Your development in the workplace is tightly linked with how safe and supported you feel in that environment. It's important to work with your HR department and event planners to ensure that non-alcoholic options are always available, making inclusivity a standard practice. Expressing your needs for a sober environment not only benefits you but also creates a more accepting culture in the workplace. Being open about your sobriety can be liberating, and you may find that it invites respect and support from colleagues who value your honesty and commitment to your health.

Career growth while maintaining your sobriety is not only possible but can also be a rewarding aspect of your recovery. As you establish your goals and work toward continuous personal and professional development, you'll realize the full potential of what you can achieve. This might involve seeking a career coach to enhance your skills, negotiate raises, or even chart a new career path. Regularly self-assessing your skills and passions and using tools like the Ikigai exercise can tailor your career trajectory to align with your recovery journey. As you gain clarity on your interests and strengths, pursue learning opportunities that fuel your creativity and drive. In doing so, you'll thrive in your current role and open yourself up to the possibility of transitions that reflect your true passions and abilities.

TIP

While openness about your recovery journey can be empowering and foster a supportive workplace environment, it is important to gauge the culture of the organization you are joining. Some companies may be less receptive due to past experiences or prevailing attitudes. Consider discussing your needs with HR or a trusted supervisor once you've established your value in the role, ensuring that your professional performance is consistently strong and reliable. This approach can help balance honesty with practicality.

BLENDING SOBRIETY AND SUCCESS: A PROFESSIONAL'S JOURNEY THROUGH RECOVERY IN THE CORPORATE WORLD WITH ALYSSE

As an established professional who embraced sobriety in 2006 at the age of thirty, I was initially reluctant to disclose my recovery journey to colleagues. As a sales and marketing department member, a significant portion of the business was conducted over libations at luncheons, after-work socials, networking events, and dinners. A strategy I adopted early in my journey was to always have a drink in hand, non-alcoholic, of course, as this typically deterred others from offering me another. For events where alcohol consumption was more prevalent, I had a planned exit strategy and a designated accountability partner, either present or accessible through my phone.

Fast-forward to a decade into my sobriety, I found myself interviewing for a position at a television station. By this point in my recovery, I had gained considerable confidence and was more open about sharing my experiences, albeit still maintaining online discretion. During these interviews, I consciously chose to advocate for myself as a person in recovery. I communicated that there might be times when I would need an extended lunch break to attend a meeting in a church basement or that I might decline or leave early from certain alcohol-centric networking events if I felt I wasn't on solid footing that day. I backed my statements with assurances that these adjustments wouldn't interfere with my professional obligations and that I remained committed to delivering exceptional work. To my delight, they offered me the position. This considered risk gave me a platform to champion change within the organization, advocating for a reevaluation of workplace drinking culture and the consistent availability of alcohol-free alternatives at all functions.

Over time, my recovery became somewhat common knowledge, and I found colleagues approaching me with queries or seeking resources, enabling me to extend my service. Service lies at the heart of my recovery, and it has been both an honor and privilege to provide support and be a reliable resource. One of my mentors once imparted a profound truth, saying, "Alysse, you have but one life; it doesn't start or end between 9 AM and 5 PM." Such wisdom underscores the futility of trying to compartmentalize personal and professional life

Enjoying happy hour and other work events

Happy hour and work events don't have to be off-limits if you approach them thoughtfully. Your involvement in the HR department and event planning can lead to the inclusion of non-alcoholic options that support your sobriety and contribute to a more inclusive work culture overall. Open communication about your sober lifestyle can be quite freeing and demonstrates your commitment to wellness and transparency.

By taking an active role in suggesting and organizing events with non-alcoholic choices, you have the power to reshape the social scene at your workplace. It's about making the gatherings comfortable for everyone, including those who choose not to drink. Your input is invaluable, as it can help create an office environment that recognizes and respects individual choices and promotes a healthier way for employees to socialize and unwind.

Furthermore, openly communicating your sobriety at work can have broader benefits beyond your well-being. Being open about your lifestyle contributes to a culture of openness where wearing a "work mask" becomes unnecessary. Your courage to be authentic might even inspire others to speak about their challenges, paving the way for a workplace that's not only about achieving goals but also about supporting each other's life choices.

Not only does integrating non-alcoholic options during work events allow you to participate fully, but it also signals to your colleagues and supervisors that you are someone who can bring about positive change. It shows that you care for the well-being of all team members, and it normalizes the idea that socializing does not have to involve alcohol to be enjoyable. Such actions could lead to broader changes in how the company handles events, which can be especially meaningful for those new to recovery and seeking a supportive environment.

Utilizing workplace support systems

The significance of utilizing workplace support systems cannot be overstressed in building a career and gaining employment, especially during recovery. Your workplace likely has various resources to support your professional growth and personal well-being. It begins with you taking a proactive approach — engage with your HR department to discuss and advocate for non-alcoholic options at work events or consult with workplace mentors on navigating career advancement opportunities. Comfort in your work environment and confidence in your professional path are both key to sustaining your sobriety and enabling your career progression.

Clear and open communication with your managers about your recovery can also be incredibly liberating and productive. It paves the way for a support system that is aware and considerate of your circumstances and might inspire policies promoting a healthier workplace culture for everyone. This transparency can help you gain access to flexible work arrangements or resources that align with your recovery goals.

REMEMBER

In your conversations with leadership, focus on how your sobriety contributes positively to your dedication and performance at work, ultimately benefiting the organization.

Beyond the immediate support systems, do not underestimate the power of career coaches and mentors in shaping your professional journey. These individuals can provide tailored advice, help you set actionable goals, and assist with skill-building essential for landing promotions or raises. Moreover, they can offer strategies for self-teaching and taking classes to facilitate a possible career change. A career coach can also help you explore new interests and passions that might align with your recovery and lead to a more fulfilling career path. It's about mapping out a trajectory that complements your newfound focus and harnesses your ambitions in recovery to their fullest potential.

Career development and advancement in recovery

As you navigate the waters of sobriety, remember that your journey is reawakening and rediscovery. Once dimmed by addiction's struggles, your ambition begins to soar in recovery, offering you the chance to harness it for your career development. Fueled by a clearer mind and a renewed spirit, this ambition can lead you to heights in your professional life that may have seemed unreachable before. Career progression is closely intertwined with your personal growth during this time. It's an opportunity to dive into uncharted territories of your interests, potentially paving the way for exciting career transitions.

During this transformative period, take the chance to reevaluate your innate abilities and interests. You're given a unique opportunity to assess what speaks to you and ignites the fire of passion within your heart. Revitalizing a sense of purpose is critical as you turn the page to a new chapter in your career. Use reflective exercises like Ikigai, which invites you to explore the convergence of what you love, what the world needs, what you can be paid for, and what you are good at. This self-inquiry can help you pinpoint a career path that brings financial stability and deeply resonates with your values and goals.

Solidifying a rewarding career while in recovery is far more than just landing a job; it's about building a life that inspires and sustains your sobriety. Open communication with your employers and HR about your recovery can foster an environment that supports your growth. Seeking professional guidance through career coaches or mentors can provide direction for skill development and strategies for discussing raises and advancement. Acknowledging and appreciating your sober journey as a critical element of your career can be both freeing and empowering, serving as a foundation for continued success and satisfaction.

Remember, your sobriety affords you a second chance at life and crafting a career that aligns with the true essence of who you are. Your time in recovery is a valuable asset: Let it guide you into a career that celebrates your strengths and passions. As you plot out your professional journey, keep an eye on the horizon of opportunities that now lie within your grasp, thanks to the clarity and purpose that recovery brings. And know that with each step forward, you build a career and solidify the fabric of a meaningful, sober livelihood.

Moving forward: Integrating career and sobriety goals

It's important to acknowledge that aligning your career goals with your sobriety is not just a task to check off — it's an ongoing, dynamic process that requires regular attention and recalibration. Your recovery is a testament to your strength and resilience and a priority; it may be the cornerstone upon which you build your professional aspirations.

As you continue your sobriety, keep in mind complacency can subtly undermine progress in your career and recovery. The perils of settling into comfort or neglecting your sobriety practices were highlighted previously and can lead to substantial setbacks (as explored in the cautionary insights of Chapter 4). It is essential to remain alert, take proactive steps, and continuously seek resources and support when required.

Let each milestone in your recovery be a stepping stone to higher ground in your career. Your experiences are unique and can provide an invaluable and irreplaceable perspective in your profession. Embrace the journey ahead with the knowledge that your sobriety doesn't limit your potential — it enhances it.

As you move forward, keep the insights from this chapter close at hand and revisit them as often as you need. Your aspirations are not merely dreams; they are the blueprints for a life of purpose, meaning, and fulfillment that you are actively building, day by sober day!

5

The Road to Long-Term Sobriety

Establish a living space that supports your sobriety

Create lifestyle changes that support long-term recovery

Use mindfulness and meditation to enhance resilience and foster connectivity

Chapter **13**

Setting the Stage for Long-Term Sobriety

I magine packing up your car and getting ready to go on a road trip adventure — not just any adventure but one that promises a renewed sense of self and the feeling of freedom with genuine fulfillment. This is precisely the *promise* of living an alcohol-free life. It's about transforming your everyday existence, not just putting a cork in the bottle. To lay the groundwork for this transformative quest, you've already started by digging deep to unearth the root causes of your substance use disorder. This could mean engaging in therapy, joining support circles, or tackling mental health concerns that dance in tandem with addiction. Remember, your recovery journey is as unique as your fingerprint — there's no one-size-fits-all map to sobriety.

In this chapter, you will look closer at establishing a sturdy platform for the future of your long-term continuous sobriety. You are constructing a bridge over troubled waters — painstaking but ultimately empowering! Healing the scars addiction has left on your life is part of this process. It involves reflecting deeply, often painfully, and striving to mend bridges where possible. This phase of your journey is not just about making amends; it's about forging a new life pattern that celebrates your choice to live soberly. It's the transition from a life of dependency to one of self-discovery and meaningful engagement — where every activity, every relationship, bears the hallmark of your commitment to sobriety.

Establishing a Solid Foundation for Recovery

Building a sustainable path to long-term sobriety often involves *redefining* your lifestyle beyond abstaining from substance use. Sobriety isn't simply a place you reach or a state to maintain; it's a continuous journey of growth and self-exploration. Consider starting your recovery by exploring the root causes of your addiction, which may include engaging in therapy, participating in support groups, and possibly addressing co-occurring mental health challenges. It's important to acknowledge that everyone's path to recovery is unique — and to celebrate milestones all along the way, whether five years of sobriety or making the daily commitment to stay sober.

As you establish the foundation for your recovery, you might find it helpful to work through the impacts that addiction has had on your life and relationships. This step could involve deep reflection and, if it feels right for you, making amends where you see fit. Your relationships are crucial in lasting happiness and addressing your past consequences; having meaningful relationships that are clear from misconduct is foundational for your sobriety and sanity!

The process of making reparations in the context of addiction recovery involves taking responsibility for past behavior and actively seeking to repair the harm caused, especially as it relates to the fallout from substance abuse. This step is a critical element of many recovery programs as it helps to heal the emotional and relational wounds stemming from addictive behaviors. Reparations usually entail a *sincere* acknowledgment of the mistakes made, an apology to those affected, and a concerted effort to remedy the harm when feasible.

An example of reparation for continuous long-term sobriety may look like this:

>> **Reflection:** Carefully consider the individuals affected and the specific harm inflicted by your actions during your use or behavior that caused harm.

>> **Preparation:** Determining the most appropriate way to approach each person affected and planning the proper form of meaningful reparation. Examples: phone calls, in-person conversations, letters, or even grave-side communication.

>> **Communication:** Initiating contact with the person who was hurt, either face-to-face or through a written message, to express understanding of the harm, apologize, and propose a way to make it right.

>> **Action:** You must take tangible measures to correct your past wrongs as much as possible, such as returning items taken, settling debts, or striving to re-establish trust and integrity.

>> **Self-forgiveness:** Recognize that making reparations is also about forgiving oneself and, moving forward, being committed to not repeating the harmful behaviors of your past.

For example, if you had caused emotional distress to a family member during your struggle with addiction, making reparations might involve a heartfelt conversation where you express your remorse, acknowledge the pain caused, and perhaps offer to attend family counseling together. If the emotional distress led to specific losses or inconveniences for the family member, you would also seek to make practical amends, such as dedicating time to help with tasks or being more *present* and supportive.

Making reparations is more than just saying you're sorry — it's about demonstrating through actions that you are earnest about mending the past and are devoted to living with integrity, which often brings healing and restoration for everyone involved.

REMEMBER

Repairing past relationships and making reparations is an integral part of healing. It involves acknowledgment, communication, and action to mend the harm done. This active process of responsibility and change is a powerful component of sustaining long-term sobriety.

Fostering relationships and cultivating new, positive habits can support your sobriety journey. Identifying activities and hobbies that bring you joy and fulfillment, independent of substances, can also contribute to developing resilient coping strategies.

The environment you create for yourself and the company you keep play significant roles in your long-term sobriety. Surrounding yourself with individuals who encourage your sober lifestyle and align with your values, such as participating in sober communities or groups with similar objectives, can be beneficial.

Building a supportive network

Surrounding yourself with sober, supportive individuals is crucial in your sobriety journey. Your support network should evolve with you, offering the necessary resources and empathy to help you navigate challenges. This network can include sober friends, support groups, and professionals who understand the importance of a sustained recovery environment. As you progress in your journey, the people around you play a pivotal role in helping maintain your sobriety. They provide companionship and accountability, serving as a mirror to reflect your progress and areas needing improvement.

Choosing the right people to be part of your support network is vital. Look for individuals who are not only sober themselves but also committed to a healthy lifestyle. Attending meetings or joining sober communities can connect you with people who share similar goals and struggles. Over time, these relationships can grow deeper, providing a reliable source of strength during times of temptation or emotional stress. Furthermore, professionals such as therapists or counselors *trained* in addiction recovery can offer insights and tools that peer support cannot, ensuring you have access to comprehensive support.

Your mental and emotional strength in sobriety increases with each day you choose to live free from alcohol or drugs. This growing strength equips you to make decisions that honor your values, such as the difficult choice to leave relationships that may be unsupportive, unsafe, or harmful to your recovery. Sobriety provides the clarity to evaluate which connections are truly beneficial to you. Be ready to reevaluate and adjust your social circle as needed because the support that serves you well may change over time. It may be essential to seek out new peers or groups that align with your present recovery phase or to distance yourself from relationships that are no longer conducive to your well-being. The aim is to nurture a network that reliably supports your journey toward lasting sobriety, sustains your emotional and psychological health, and fortifies your ability to overcome the complexities of maintaining sobriety.

TIP

Think of your support network as a garden. Just as gardens require periodic weeding and new plants to thrive, your social landscape also needs tending. Regularly assess the health of your relationships. Cultivate connections with sober, healthy-minded individuals and seek out support groups or professional guidance where you can share and learn in a community with common ground.

Developing healthy coping mechanisms

As you transition from old habits, it's essential to identify and understand your triggers, aka *spark points*. Spark points are those moments or situations that can prompt a response that might challenge your sobriety. They are the catalysts for emotional or physical reactions that may lead to cravings or discomfort. Recognizing and understanding your spark points is integral to the journey to long-term sobriety.

REMEMBER

In Chapter 10, we explored identifying personal spark points and their significance in your recovery process. You learned that being mindful of these spark points and developing strategies to navigate them is essential for maintaining your sobriety.

As you continue to build your resilience, remember that everyone's experience with spark points is unique. They can be tied to specific emotional states, environmental factors, or stressors. As you progress in your recovery, the spark points you once faced may evolve or change, and new ones will emerge. Continuously adapting your coping strategies to address these changes is crucial for lasting sobriety.

Once you know your spark points, the next step is to seek appropriate therapies or support systems that prevent cross-addictions. Cross-addiction occurs when quitting one addiction leads to developing another. To avoid this, integrate therapies like cognitive-behavioral therapy, mindfulness, or even peer support groups that focus on comprehensive addiction recovery. The goal is not merely to replace one unhealthy habit with another but to foster positive change in your lifestyle and behavior patterns.

Align your lifestyle with your commitment to sobriety. Make conscious decisions that reinforce your coping strategies. For instance, maintaining a regular exercise routine can help manage stress and improve mental health. Additionally, curating a social circle supporting your sober lifestyle can provide encouragement and accountability. By carefully structuring your environment to minimize stress and sparks and actively choosing practices that promote your well-being, you create a fertile ground for sustainable recovery.

Following is a list of healthy coping mechanisms:

>> **Mindfulness techniques:** Practice meditation, deep breathing, or yoga to ground yourself and manage stress.

>> **Physical activity:** Regularly exercise, such as walking, swimming, or attending fitness classes, to release tension and improve mood.

>> **Creative outlets:** Channel your energy into creative activities like painting, writing, or playing music to express emotions and reduce anxiety.

>> **Structured routine:** Create a daily schedule that includes time for self-care, work, and leisure to bring stability and predictability to your life.

- **Hobbies:** Take up new or rediscover old hobbies that engage your interest and attention and provide a sense of accomplishment and joy.

- **Journaling:** Keep a journal to track your feelings, spark points, and coping strategies. This will help you reflect and adapt as needed.

- **Nutrition:** Focus on a balanced diet that supports physical health and mental clarity, which can positively affect your emotional state.

- **Educational resources:** Read books, attend workshops, or listen to podcasts about sobriety and recovery to gather knowledge and stay motivated.

- **Volunteering:** Give back to your community through volunteer work, which can provide a sense of purpose and connectedness.

- **Professional help for cross-addiction:** If faced with cross-addiction risk, seek specialized assistance to address and prevent it.

- **Environmental management:** Organize your living and working spaces to reduce stressors and remove reminders of past substance use.

- **Assertiveness training:** Learn to communicate your needs effectively and set boundaries to protect your sobriety.

When you implement these coping mechanisms, you create a robust framework for handling life's challenges without compromising your commitment to sobriety. Each strategy contributes to building a comprehensive approach to maintaining your recovery and enhancing your overall well-being.

Creating a sober living environment

Your living environment is a fundamental aspect of your journey toward long-term sobriety. It should serve as a sanctuary, free from substances and influences that could jeopardize your recovery. Ensuring your home environment is safe, stable, and supportive involves more than just removing temptations; it's about creating a space that reinforces your daily habits and routines conducive to a sober lifestyle. Prioritize organizing and maintaining an orderly space that helps minimize stress and promote mental clarity.

Understanding recovery's neurobiological underpinnings can illuminate your journey toward sustained sobriety. In Chapter 10, we discussed the importance of your living environment in supporting your sobriety. It's not just about removing temptations; it's about creating a space that promotes the balance of essential neurotransmitters — particularly dopamine and serotonin — in your brain.

Dopamine is often referred to as the "feel-good" neurotransmitter. It's associated with the pleasure system of the brain, providing feelings of enjoyment and reinforcement to motivate us to perform certain activities proactively yet it can reinforce maladaptive behaviors. Your sobriety can benefit from natural dopamine boosts, which may result from rewarding activities such as exercise, hobbies, and meaningful social interactions.

Serotonin, on the other hand, is key to your sense of well-being and happiness. Beyond its mood-lifting effects, serotonin helps regulate sleep patterns, appetite, and impulse control — all critical for stable recovery. Maintaining a well-balanced diet rich in tryptophan — an amino acid precursor to serotonin — can support your emotional states and aid in reducing cravings.

Harmonizing your space for neurobiology

In your pursuit of a balanced life, it's crucial to consider how your environment can support or hinder the regulation of these neurotransmitters. Here are some practical ways to create a living space that encourages stable dopamine and serotonin levels:

>> **Natural light and serenity:** Sunlight naturally enhances serotonin production. Create a space with plenty of natural light and areas dedicated to relaxation and meditation to support serotonin levels.

>> **Organization and clarity:** A cluttered environment can lead to a cluttered mind. Keeping your living space tidy can reduce stress, allowing dopamine pathways to function without additional strain.

>> **Social interactions:** Cultivate a social environment that encourages positive interactions. Meaningful conversations and connections can stimulate dopamine release through social bonding.

>> **Nutrition station:** Set up a kitchen space that invites healthy eating. Foods that contain tryptophan, omega-3 fatty acids, and antioxidants can support serotonin production and overall brain health.

>> **Activity zones:** Designate areas for physical activity, art, or music. Engaging in these activities can boost dopamine and provide an outlet for self-expression and skill development.

REMEMBER

Your living environment plays a crucial role in reinforcing the healthy habits contributing to your recovery. By aligning your space with the needs of your neurobiology, you create a supportive backdrop for the intricate work of maintaining sobriety.

You can also refer to Chapter 5, where we discussed genetic factors and environmental influences, to see how a supportive living environment can interact with your biological predispositions to foster recovery. Chapter 15 explores coping mechanisms that complement these neurobiological strategies, providing an even more comprehensive approach to building resilience in your sober life.

TIP

Your path to recovery is as much about nurturing your mind as it is about breaking free from substances. Understanding these neurobiological principles and sculpting your environment empowers your brain's chemistry to support your sobriety goals.

Identifying warning signs

Understanding the warning signs that lead to relapse is the first crucial step in crafting your comprehensive relapse prevention plan. This process demands deep self-awareness and a willingness to delve into your past behaviors and environments.

By exploring these areas, you recognize the patterns and circumstances that have previously led to setbacks.

Now, let's identify specific behaviors and situations that serve as spark points — the catalysts for relapse — and understand the corresponding warning signs of falling back into old, unhealthy habits. You will need a journal or digital document, a writing utensil or digital input method, and a comfortable, distraction-free environment.

Follow these instructions:

1. Find a quiet space where you can think without interruption.

2. Prepare your journal or digital document for taking notes.

3. Center yourself with a few deep breaths to focus on the task at hand.

4. Conduct a behavioral analysis:

- Write the heading "If I do X" at the top of your journal or document.

- Reflect on past behaviors that have led to adverse outcomes or feelings.

5. Identify your spark points:

- Under this heading, create three columns: "Behavior," "Warning Signs," and "If-Then Scenarios."

- These might include actions, thoughts, or emotional states that have previously contributed to unhealthy choices.

6. Fill in the columns as follows:

- **Behavior:**

  - Reflect on past behaviors that have led to adverse outcomes or feelings.

  - List the behaviors you recognize as problematic or potentially risky.

- **Warning signs:**
  - For each behavior listed, identify accompanying warning signs indicating you're approaching or engaging in a spark point.
  - Warning signs can be physical (such as increased heart rate), emotional (such as feeling anxious), or cognitive (such as justifying risky behavior).
- **If-then scenarios:**
  - Using your "Behavior" list, create if-then scenarios that depict a causal relationship between the behavior and its outcome.
  - For example, "If I start isolating myself, then I might start feeling lonely and consider reaching out to old substance-using friends."

5. **Identify your spark points:**

  - List behaviors you recognize as problematic or potentially risky.
  - These might include actions, thoughts, or emotional states that have previously contributed to unhealthy choices.

6. **Recognize your warning signs:**

  - For each behavior listed, identify accompanying warning signs, indicating you're approaching or engaging in a spark point.
  - Warning signs can be physical (such as increased heart rate), emotional (such as feeling anxious), or cognitive (such as justifying risky behavior).

7. **Construct "if-then" scenarios:**

  - Using your "If I do X" list, create if-then scenarios that depict a causal relationship between the behavior and its outcome.
  - For example, "If I start isolating myself, then I might start feeling lonely and consider reaching out to old substance-using friends."

8. Strategize healthy reactions:

- For each if-then scenario, write down a healthy counter-action or coping strategy.

- Ensure these strategies are practical and can be implemented immediately upon recognizing the warning signs.

9. Rehearse your responses:

- Visualize each if-then scenario and mentally rehearse your healthy reaction.

- Consider role-playing these scenarios with a trusted support person to practice your responses.

10. Consolidate your plan:

- Gather all the "if-then" scenarios and corresponding healthy reactions into one comprehensive document.

- Title this document "My Spark Points and Warning Signs Action Plan."

11. Reflect on the exercise and how it made you feel:

- You've taken a proactive step in understanding and managing your behaviors by identifying your spark points and corresponding warning signs. Review and update your action plan regularly or whenever you notice changes in your habits or emotional state.

Table 13-1 shows an example of what a completed action plan might look like.

TABLE 13-1   ## Identifying Spark Points

Behavior	Warning Signs	If-Then Scenarios
Isolating myself	Feeling lonely Justifying risky behavior	If I start isolating myself, then I might start feeling lonely and consider reaching out to old substance-using friends.
Staying up late	Increased heart rate Feeling anxious	If I stay up late, then I might feel more stressed and crave alcohol to relax.
Avoiding social events	Feeling anxious Negative thoughts	If I avoid social events, then I might feel more isolated and turn to old habits.

REMEMBER

This exercise aims not to criticize yourself for past behaviors but to empower yourself with the knowledge and strategies you need to maintain your recovery. Keep your action plan accessible and use it as a guide whenever you encounter spark points.

By knowing what specific signs precede a relapse — be it increased stress, specific social scenarios, or emotional upheavals — you can implement strategies to tackle these issues early on. Whether it's reaching out to a sponsor, attending more frequent support group meetings, or practicing mindfulness, acting on the early warning signs can help prevent a full-blown relapse. Consequently, your relapse prevention plan becomes a dynamic living tool that adapts to your evolving needs and challenges in sobriety.

Crafting a Comprehensive Relapse Prevention Plan

Creating a comprehensive relapse prevention plan is crucial in maintaining long-term sobriety. This plan begins with acknowledging the *potential* for relapse, making it a proactive approach rather than a reactive one. You and your family or partners *must* discuss openly the possibility of relapse and set mutual expectations. Identifying specific *spark points* and early warning signs that may threaten your sobriety is essential. Understanding these can provide clear strategies for dealing with high-risk situations.

In your prevention plan, it's essential to incorporate strategies that include effective communication with your support network. Whether this involves daily check-ins with a sponsor or support group or having a system in place for reaching out during times of high stress, these steps can offer significant protective benefits. Also, consider legal or structural responses like involving police or healthcare professionals, if necessary, as part of a safety plan to handle extremely challenging scenarios. Setting hard boundaries with yourself and others can prevent scenarios that might lead to relapse.

Building your personal relapse prevention blueprint

Here, you'll create a dynamic and comprehensive relapse prevention plan as your roadmap for continuous long-term sobriety. You'll need a journal or digital document, a pen or typing device, and a quiet place.

Follow these instructions:

1. **Reflection and acknowledgment:**

- Begin with a moment of reflection on your journey so far.

- Acknowledge the potential for relapse as a part of the recovery process.

- Write down your commitment to a proactive, not reactive, approach to preventing relapse.

2. **Communication strategy:**

- Plan how you will communicate with your support network.

- Decide on the frequency of check-ins with your sponsor or support group.

- Outline clear steps for reaching out during high-stress situations.

3. **Spark points:**

- List your known spark points and early warning signs that may threaten your sobriety.

- For each spark point, write a strategy to counteract or cope with it.

4. **Legal and structural responses:**

- Consider extreme scenarios where involving authorities or healthcare professionals may be necessary.

- Create a safety plan with steps to handle these challenges.

- Determine what legal or structural responses you're comfortable with and include these in your plan.

5. **Boundary setting:**

   - Define hard boundaries with yourself and those around you to prevent high-risk scenarios.

   - Document specific scenarios where you need to enforce these boundaries.

6. **Regular review:**

   - Schedule monthly reviews of your relapse prevention plan to ensure it remains relevant.

   - Adjust strategies in response to personal growth or changing circumstances.

7. **Contingency planning:**

   - Develop contingency plans with clear indicators for when to seek additional assistance.

   - Outline potential responses or consequences if recovery goals are not met.

8. **Your blueprint:**

   - Compile all the elements into a structured relapse prevention plan.

   - Ensure it's accessible by keeping a physical copy or storing it digitally where it can be easily retrieved.

Once you have drafted your relapse prevention blueprint, share it with a trusted support network member. This can be your sponsor, a therapist, or a close family member. Their feedback can provide valuable insights and help you refine your plan. Keep this blueprint as a living document that grows and adapts with you throughout your sobriety journey.

REMEMBER

Your relapse prevention plan is your blueprint for resilient, continuous sobriety. It's a testament to your dedication to your recovery and a guide that empowers you to navigate the challenges.

Implementing strategies for high-risk situations

Navigating the sometimes treacherous path of sobriety, you will inevitably encounter moments that test the very fabric of who you are and who you are becoming; these are known as high-risk situations. Recognizing your unique spark points is a vital piece of this complex puzzle. With this knowledge in hand, you can construct and enforce robust personal boundaries, thus granting you a shield of empowerment against the allure of old habits. Take, for instance, the stress-inducing atmosphere of a demanding job that might once have coaxed you into unhealthy coping mechanisms. Establishing and insisting upon a clear delineation between professional and personal time and advocating for supportive measures within your workplace is not just beneficial — it's essential.

Fortifying against high-risk situations

In this section, you'll enhance your resilience in high-risk situations by equipping yourself with clear strategies and an actionable plan to protect your sobriety when faced with severe challenges. You'll need a detailed list of personal triggers (from previous exercises), a journal or digital document for creating your high-risk plan, and access to your support network's contact information.

Follow these instructions:

1. Defining high-risk situations:

- Review and list specific scenarios that you consider high risk for triggering a relapse.

- Be explicit about the settings, individuals involved, and feelings these situations evoke.

2. Setting boundaries:

- For each high-risk situation, outline practical boundaries to prevent or minimize exposure.

- Determine your steps if someone or something crosses these boundaries.

3. Creating your safety protocols:

- Develop a protocol for those potential instances where a trigger could escalate into a direct threat to your sobriety.

- Include steps involving law enforcement or other authorities, detailing under what circumstances and how these resources will be contacted.

4. Activating your support network:

- Name specific individuals or groups that constitute your support network.
- Develop a communication plan for connecting with them during high-risk situations, including phone calls, texts, or meeting arrangements.

5. Practicing and rehearsing:

- Role-play high-risk scenarios with a trusted member of your support network.
- Rehearse implementing your boundaries and safety protocols until you feel confident in your responses.

6. Documenting your action plan:

- Compile the identified high-risk situations, boundaries, safety protocols, and support network strategies into a comprehensive plan.
- Title the document "My High-Risk Situations Sobriety Shield."

Confirm that your "sobriety shield" plan is actionable and realistic. Keep it readily accessible and review it regularly with your support network to ensure its effectiveness. In moments of peace, visualize yourself successfully handling high-risk situations, reinforcing your strategies.

REMEMBER

Being prepared for high-risk situations is an act of self-compassion and strength. Your sobriety is of utmost importance, and having a plan is not an overreaction — it's a courageous step toward safeguarding the life you are building. Use the sobriety shield as a testament to your commitment to recovery and as a reminder that you have the power and support to maintain your path, no matter the challenges that arise.

Regularly reviewing and adjusting the plan

After setting up a relapse prevention plan, it's vital not just to leave it in the back drawer and forget about it. Continuous sobriety *requires* a proactive approach, regularly reviewing and adjusting your plan. This adjustment might be necessary as you grow emotionally, encounter new spark points, or when significant life changes occur. Keeping your plan dynamic ensures it remains relevant and effective in supporting your sobriety journey.

Recognizing that you are not the same person you were at the start of your sobriety journey is crucial to your continued success. Your needs, challenges, and the environments you navigate will also change as you evolve. This means that the coping mechanisms and strategies you initially put in place might not be as effective in the face of new challenges. Monthly, quarterly, and even yearly reviews of your plan can allow you to identify what's working and what's not, allowing for timely adjustments before small issues threaten your sobriety.

Beyond personal evolution, life's unpredictability requires flexibility in your relapse prevention plan. Whether transitioning to a new job, dealing with family issues, or moving to a new area, these changes can unsettle your routine and expose you to new risks. Regularly updating your plan to reflect these life changes enhances your resilience against relapse. Keep in constant communication with your support network about these updates, ensuring they can offer the most appropriate support when needed. This ongoing revision and reinforcement of your plan is a testament to your commitment to a sober and healthier lifestyle.

TIP

Keep your relapse prevention plan alive by thinking of your relapse prevention plan as a living document — one that breathes, grows, and evolves with you. Schedule regular audits of your plan to ensure that it remains a robust support in your recovery. Embrace these reviews not as a chore, but as opportunities to renew your commitment to sobriety and to fine-tune your defenses against the challenges that lie ahead.

REMEMBER

A plan that adapts is a plan that sustains.

The Journey of Sustained and Continuous Sobriety

Sustained and continuous sobriety is not simply a matter of abstaining from substances; it's a profound journey of personal transformation that requires commitment, awareness, and a willingness to change daily. As you reflect on this journey, recognize that the road to long-term sobriety can vary significantly from one individual to another.

Developing and refining coping mechanisms is an ongoing aspect of the sobriety journey. This involves identifying habits that no longer serve your best interests and implementing new strategies to manage life's stresses and challenges. Be vigilant about cross-addictions and make a conscientious effort to confront and modify these behaviors. Acknowledging the possibility of relapse is important, and crafting a comprehensive relapse prevention plan should be a priority. Such a plan includes identifying potential triggers, establishing clear boundaries, and discussing strategies with your support network to ensure you're prepared for high-risk situations.

Long-term sobriety is not a linear path but a continuous evolution of your habits and mindset. You must be willing to adapt your strategies for handling life's stresses and unexpected challenges. *Self-preservation* in this context means prioritizing your mental and emotional health and ensuring healthy boundaries and coping mechanisms. It is vital to regularly review and adjust your relapse prevention strategies as circumstances and personal growth dictate. Embracing adaptability and preserving your well-being are key elements in indefinitely maintaining a sober life.

TIP

Self-preservation in recovery is not a selfish act; it's a necessary measure. It *requires* you to be vigilant about protecting your mental, emotional, and physical health. Adapting your defenses to align with your current reality ensures that the safeguards you rely on are as strong as they can be.

Change, growth, and new experiences are a part of life — and your sobriety strategy should reflect this. The adjustment process is not about overhauling the core of your plan but fine-tuning it. This might include incorporating new self-care techniques, setting fresh boundaries, or seeking additional support. By doing so, you fortify your commitment to a sober lifestyle that's not only manageable but thriving.

REMEMBER

Your sobriety journey is yours, and so, too, must be your approach. Embrace the role of adaptability and self-preservation as your guides. They are the guardians of your well-being and the architects of your resilience. As you continue to grow in your recovery, let these principles light your path and remind you that your commitment to sobriety is not just a phase — *it's a way of life.*

Chapter **14**

Lifestyle Changes for Lasting Sobriety

E mbracing a life of recovery is akin to reshaping your existence from the ground up, and you can do this and redo this at one year sober or twenty-five years sober. Lasting sobriety is a commitment to leaving behind old patterns and carving out a new path, where the ideals of physical well-being, mental clarity, and emotional growth guide your journey. It might not be hyperbolic to say that this is a rebirth, a chance to redefine your narrative and the role that sobriety plays within it.

As you unfold the pages of this chapter, you will have the opportunity to explore the bedrock of such a transformation — lifestyle changes for lasting sobriety. This isn't about temporary adjustments but rather the cultivation of a life steeped in the values and routines that support your recovery. From nurturing your physical health through nutrition and exercise to fostering mental resilience through mindfulness and stress management, this chapter equips you with the strategies to survive and thrive in sobriety.

Your recovery isn't a destination but a *dynamic, living process* that evolves as you do. Thus, as you step into this chapter, remember that these aren't just changes but investments in a foundation that will support the life you choose to build every day.

Creating a Sober-Friendly Daily Routine

Establishing a daily routine tailored to support your sobriety can be a transformative tool in your recovery journey. A consistent routine helps normalize your day-to-day activities and reinforces stability and predictability, which is comforting when navigating life's challenges. By waking up and going to bed at the same time each day, you create a rhythm that your body and mind can rely on, reducing stress and minimizing the risks of idle time that might lead to temptations. Incorporating proper nutrition into your daily schedule is equally essential.

A balanced diet that includes regular meals and healthy snacks can prevent fluctuations in blood sugar, which are often responsible for mood swings and cravings.

Amino acids, the building blocks of proteins, are pivotal in producing neurotransmitters, which regulate mood and cravings. For instance, the amino acid tyrosine is a precursor to dopamine, a neurotransmitter that's often depleted in early recovery due to substance use. You can naturally boost your dopamine levels, enhancing well-being and motivation by incorporating foods rich in tyrosine, such as chicken, eggs, fish, and certain dairy products.

Similarly, tryptophan, found in turkey, nuts, seeds, and tofu, is essential for the production of serotonin, often referred to as the "happiness hormone." Ensuring you get enough tryptophan can help stabilize your mood and improve sleep, which is often disrupted in recovery.

In your daily routine, consider starting the day with a breakfast high in protein to kickstart your neurotransmitter production. Midday meals and snacks should include a balance of complex carbohydrates, lean proteins, and healthy fats to sustain your energy levels and keep your blood sugar stable. This will help avoid the mood swings and cravings that might otherwise jeopardize your sobriety.

Remember to hydrate, too; adequate water intake is vital for all bodily functions, including the efficient use of nutrients. And don't forget about the importance of consistently timing your meals to stabilize your body's body's rhythms further.

Physical activity, as part of your daily routine, not only helps release endorphins but also aids in regulating your body's stress response. This can be particularly beneficial in managing any feelings of unease or urges that might arise.

TIP

Ensure that your routine includes plenty of opportunities for relaxation and reflection. Practices like meditation, deep-breathing exercises, or journaling can all serve as valuable tools for mental clarity and emotional regulation, anchoring your commitment to a wholesome and sober lifestyle. Integrating these elements into your daily schedule will help create a holistic approach to your recovery, supporting both your physical and mental health on the road to long-term sobriety.

Follow these instructions to create a sober-friendly daily routine:

1. Fill out this worksheet daily to maintain a sober-friendly routine.

2. Adjust times and activities based on your preferences and schedule.

3. Use the reflection section to remind yourself of your progress.

4. If you face challenges, refer to your coping strategies and reach out to your support system.

   - **Morning routine:**
     - Wake-up time: _____
     - Morning self-care activities:
       1. Exercise (type and duration): _____
       2. Meditation/mindfulness practice (duration): _____
       3. Nutritional breakfast choice: _____

- **Work/study schedule:**
  - Start time: _____
  - Key tasks for today:
    1. _____
    2. _____
    3. _____
  - Break times (for snacks, walk, reflection): _____
- **Afternoon check-in:**
  - Current mood: _____
  - Stress level (1-10): _____
  - Coping strategy if my stress level is higher than 5: _____

4. **Evening activities:**
   - Sober social activity: _____
   - Dinner plan (healthy meal choice): _____
   - Evening relaxation practice: _____

5. **Nighttime routine:**
   - Preparing for tomorrow (clothes, meals, schedule): _____
   - Sleep hygiene practice (screen time, reading, meditation): _____
   - Bedtime: _____

6. **Reflection:**
   - Favorite part of today: _____
   - Something you're grateful For: _____
   - A goal for tomorrow: _____

7. **Sobriety tracker:**
   - Days/months/years sober: _____
   - Feelings about sobriety today: _____
   - Sobriety support contact (if needed): _____

Figure 14-1 is an example of a sober–friendly daily routine worksheet.

SOBER-FRIENDLY DAILY ROUTINE WORKSHEET

MORNING ROUTINE:

WAKE-UP TIME:

TODAY'S MORNING SELF-CARE ACTIVITIES:

- _____
- _____
- _____

WORK/STUDY SCHEDULE/TASKS:

START TIME:

KEY TASKS FOR TODAY:

- _____
- _____
- _____

TAKE A BREAK (SNACK, WALK, REFLECTION):

_____
_____
_____
_____

AFTERNOON CHECK-IN:

CURRENT MOOD: _____

STRESS LEVEL (1-10): _____

COPING STRATEGY IF STRESS IF HIGHER THAN 5:

_____
_____

FIGURE 14-1:
Sober-
friendly daily
routine
worksheet.

SOBER-FRIENDLY DAILY ROUTINE WORKSHEET

EVENING ACTIVITIES:

TODAY'S EVENING ACTIVITIES:

● _____

● _____

● _____

NIGHT-TIME ROUTINE:

PREPARING FOR TOMORROW (CLOTHES, MEALS, SCHEDULE):

_____

_____

SLEEP HYGIENE PRACTICE (SCREEN TIME, READING, MEDITATION):

_____

_____

BEDTIME: _____

REFLECTION:

FAVORITE PART OF TODAY, GRATEFUL FOR, GOAL FOR TOMORROW:

_____

_____

_____

_____

SOBRIETY TRACKER:

DAYS/MONTHS/YEARS SOBER: _____

FEELINGS ABOUT SOBRIETY TODAY:

_____

SOBRIETY SUPPORT CONTACT: _____

FIGURE 14-1:
(Continued)

Sleep and sobriety

Establishing a consistent wake-up and bedtime routine is critical to supporting your journey of long-term sobriety and getting an adequate amount of good quality sleep. A regular sleep schedule helps stabilize your internal clock, enhancing mood and energy levels throughout the day. This routine minimizes the unpredictability in your life, which can often lead to stress and, consequently, temptations to relapse. By prioritizing specific times to wake up and go to bed each day, you build a stable foundation for your daily activities, significantly aiding your sobriety journey.

Starting and ending your day at the same time helps develop other sobriety-supporting habits and routines. Morning rituals like meditation, exercise, or reading can fit well into this structure, creating a proactive start to your day that focuses on well-being. Night routines can involve activities like journaling or planning the next day that calm the mind and prepare it for rest. Embracing these habits consistently can transform them into essential components of your sobriety toolkit.

This structured approach keeps your physical body in sync and provides a psychological framework that supports sobriety. When you know what to expect at the start and end of each day, you decrease anxiety and increase your ability to handle challenges without resorting to old behaviors. Establishing and maintaining a regular sleep schedule is a foundational step in crafting a lifestyle that nurtures and sustains long-term sobriety.

Scientific evidence supports that quality sleep is critical for various aspects of brain function, including cognitive performance, emotional regulation, and mental health. Sleep facilitates the clearance of metabolites from the brain, including beta-amyloid, which accumulates during waking hours. Adequate sleep also plays a crucial role in fostering neuroplasticity, the brain's ability to adapt and rewire itself — a vital factor in recovery and long-term sobriety. Solidifying your wake-up and bedtime routine, accompanied by restorative sleep, is an investment in your brain health, emotional balance, and, ultimately, recovery.

Incorporating healthy meals and snacks into daily life

Nourishing yourself with balanced, nutritious food choices is essential in fostering resilience and continuity in your recovery. The role of a nutrient-dense diet, punctuated by amino acids and high-quality proteins, cannot be overstated when it comes to promoting strength and gaining psychological stability. Proteins are not just nutrients; they're the precursors to neurotransmitters that regulate your mood and neural processes, integral to a well-functioning brain and a balanced emotional state.

In your quest for wellness, it's important to remember that these amino acids and proteins are more than mere sustenance; they're the very materials your body uses to rebuild and replenish itself. By consciously including them in your meals and various other healthy foods, you're laying the groundwork for a better body and mind to handle the rigors of sober living. Your dietary choices directly influence the biochemical landscape of your brain, impacting your ability to think clearly, manage stress, and retain control over your impulses and decisions.

To ensure your body receives the nutrition it deserves, focus on integrating a variety of foods into your meals, emphasizing amino-rich proteins such as lean meats, fish, eggs, and legumes. These proteins support the repair of tissues and the production of enzymes and hormones that are critical for maintaining clear thinking. Complement these with various fruits, vegetables, and whole grains to create a nutrient-dense diet that fuels recovery.

REMEMBER

Every meal is a stepping stone on your path to recovery. Through mindful nutrition, you have the power to shape not only your physical health but also your mental fortitude. Embrace the knowledge that the proteins and amino acids you consume do more than satisfy hunger — they play a profound role in repairing your body and fortifying your mind. By choosing foods that are rich in essential nutrients, you're actively contributing to the stability and clarity needed for a sober lifestyle.

Remember that your brain relies on a delicate balance of neurotransmitters, and what you eat directly contributes to this balance. Eating healthy is not just about eating healthy; it's about feeding your recovery, one meal at a time. Make a conscious effort to include a variety of amino acid-rich proteins in your diet, and don't forget to complement them with a colorful array of fruits, vegetables, and whole grains for comprehensive nutrition.

Your diet is a powerful ally in managing your well-being. The daily fuel supports your body's recovery and the clarity and control you seek in your thoughts and emotions. Let your meals be a testament to your dedication to sobriety, a symbol of your resolve to rebuild and rejuvenate every aspect of yourself.

In addition to protein intake, avoiding large gaps between meals is essential to help stabilize blood sugar levels and prevent cravings and mood swings. Regular nourishment is critical — aim to incorporate snacks that balance protein, carbohydrates, and healthy fats, allowing for sustained energy and mood regulation throughout the day.

Understanding the interplay between nutrition and emotional health is central to your recovery. Inconsistent eating patterns and imbalanced meals can trigger fluctuations in blood sugar, which may lead to feelings of anxiety, irritability, and depression. These states can increase the risk of relapse. Strategically planned meals and snacks that provide a balance of nutrients empower you to moderate your mood and fortify your commitment to sobriety.

Invest time in meal planning and preparation to harness the benefits of a nutritious diet. Set aside weekly moments to organize your meals, ensuring you have ready access to the foods supporting your recovery. This practice minimizes stress and upholds your daily dedication to maintaining your sobriety. Each mindful choice at the dining table is a pledge to a healthier, more resilient you, paving the way for a successful, sober lifestyle.

TIP

When optimizing your diet for recovery, consider hiring a professional nutritionist specializing in this area. A nutritionist with experience in recovery can tailor your meal plan to your specific needs, ensuring you receive the correct balance of amino acids, proteins, and other nutrients essential for restoring your health. They can simplify the process, saving you time and money in the long run by preventing the trial and error that often accompanies self-guided nutritional changes. With their guidance, you'll find it easier to make informed choices and establish sustainable eating habits that support your journey to lasting sobriety.

Here's a sample plan that focuses on foods rich in amino acids, which are vital for neurotransmitter production, mood regulation, and overall brain function:

» Day 1:

- **Breakfast:** Scrambled eggs with spinach and whole-grain toast. Eggs are an excellent source of essential amino acids, and spinach provides additional nutrients that support brain health.

- **Snack:** Greek yogurt with mixed berries and a sprinkle of chia seeds. Greek yogurt is high in protein, and the berries add a dose of antioxidants.

- **Lunch:** Grilled chicken breast salad with mixed greens, cherry tomatoes, avocado, and a vinaigrette dressing. Chicken is a lean protein that's rich in tryptophan, while avocado delivers healthy fats.

- **Snack:** A handful of almonds and an apple. Almonds are a good source of protein and healthy fats.

- **Dinner:** Baked salmon with quinoa and steamed broccoli. Salmon is full of omega-3 fatty acids, and quinoa is a complete protein, which means it contains all essential amino acids.

» Day 2:

- **Breakfast:** Protein-packed smoothie with plant protein, fresh berries, almond milk, and a tablespoon of almond butter.

- **Snack:** A hard-boiled egg and a few carrot sticks with hummus. The egg provides protein, and the hummus is rich in chickpea amino acids.

- **Lunch:** Turkey breast wrap using romaine lettuce as a wrap, filled with tomatoes, onions, and mustard. Turkey is another excellent source of protein.

- **Snack:** Sliced pear with a ricotta cheese dollop and a sprinkle of walnuts. The smooth, creamy ricotta offers a gentle, high-quality protein on the stomach, while the pear provides a sweet touch and a source of dietary fiber. Walnuts add a satisfying crunch and are rich in omega-3 fatty acids, which are beneficial for brain health.

- **Dinner:** Lentil soup with a side of whole-grain bread. Lentils are a great plant-based protein and rich in fiber and minerals.

REMEMBER

It's essential to include a variety of protein sources to ensure you're getting a full range of essential amino acids in your diet. Try to eat at regular intervals to maintain stable blood sugar levels, which can help manage cravings. Hydration is also crucial for overall health, so drink plenty of water daily. If you're unsure about your specific nutritional needs, consider consulting a nutritionist specializing in recovery for personalized advice.

Prioritizing regular physical activity in daily routine

Incorporating a consistent schedule of exercise into your lifestyle is pivotal to your journey of recovery from alcoholism and addiction. This practice offers multifaceted advantages, offering clear physical benefits and playing a significant role in recuperating and fortifying your brain's health. Begin with accessible activities that you can weave seamlessly into your routine, like stretching each morning or taking brisk walks. These acts are the building blocks of a rewarding regimen that can evolve with you over time.

Consistency in your physical activity is a linchpin in this process. It's crucial for tempering stress and regulating your mood — two elements that, if left unchecked, could jeopardize your hard-won sobriety. Your commitment to regular movement can act as both a shield and a foundation, protecting your progress and enhancing your overall quality of life.

Regular physical activity is crucial in rebalancing your brain's dopamine levels. During substance use, dopamine is released in excessive amounts, creating an association between the substance and pleasure that can overpower natural rewards. In recovery, as you abstain from substance use, your brain's dopamine production normalizes. Exercise can help repair the reward circuitry by providing a healthy and natural boost to dopamine levels. This increase in dopamine is essential because it compensates for the deficit that occurs upon cessation of substance use, and it does so in a way that enhances your overall well-being rather than detracting from it.

REMEMBER

Setting realistic fitness goals tailored to your preferences and physical condition is key. The activity should inspire and excite you, whether it's choosing cycling, swimming, or weight lifting. Ensure that your goals are achievable and allow room for gradual progression in intensity and duration. Celebrate your milestones — every sweat session is a step toward reinforcing your commitment to sobriety. Regularly engaging in these activities helps build endurance and physical strength and instills a sense of accomplishment and self-worth.

Socializing and Networking in Sober Circles

Socializing within sober communities is vital for your recovery. It offers you camaraderie and the accountability of peers with shared experiences. Search for activities that align with your goals, like recovery meetings or sports leagues for those in recovery. These environments provide not just fun but also reinforce your commitment to sobriety.

Building connections with others in recovery allows for a special kind of support. Active participation in groups and workshops fosters an empathetic and reinforcing network. Develop friendships with those who respect and support your sober lifestyle by engaging in activities that bolster your joint dedication to sobriety. A strong, sober social circle helps combat recovery's potential isolation.

Nurturing supportive friendships in recovery involves more than just casual meetings; it requires a concerted effort to cultivate relationships that positively influence your sobriety. Choose friends who respect your lifestyle choices and encourage your growth. Plan sober-friendly activities together, such as hiking, attending art classes, or cooking meals. These interactions strengthen your bonds and support your mutual commitment to sobriety. Moreover, being part of a community dedicated to sober living helps mitigate feelings of isolation and loneliness, which are often encountered in recovery.

Sober social events and activities

You might find that socializing while maintaining sobriety requires some creativity. Engaging in sober-friendly activities like attending concerts, joining hiking gatherings, or going to sober parties allows you to enjoy life without the interference of substances. Planning events that do not center around alcohol or drugs not only keeps you safe but also reinforces your commitment to sobriety.

Engaging in sober social events and activities is an enriching part of the recovery journey. Consider trying out some of the following activities:

>> Host a game night with a selection of board games and puzzles for an entertaining evening.

>> Organize or join an escape room group to enjoy the thrill and camaraderie that comes with teamwork.

>> Participate in outdoor adventures such as hiking, rock climbing, or kayaking, offering a natural high and a sense of accomplishment! Everyone loves a first time!

>> Engage in creative workshops like painting, pottery, or writing, which can be therapeutic and provide a channel for expressing emotions.

>> Explore volunteer opportunities within your community that can give you a sense of purpose and community connection.

>> Attend or organize sober parties where everyone is on the same page about not drinking, ensuring a comfortable and pressure-free environment.

>> Join a sports league or fitness class specifically designed for individuals in recovery; this will also aid in physical well-being. A sober yoga class is spectacular for your body and spirit!

>> Discover local cultural events, such as theater productions, art exhibits, or music concerts focusing on the arts rather than alcohol.

Keep track of the activities that bring you the most joy and fulfill-ment. You can maintain a social activity tracker to gauge which events lead to a higher sense of connection and overall mood improvement. This approach not only offers you diversion and enjoyment but also reinforces your sober lifestyle and educates others about the joys and possibilities of living alcohol-free.

Don't underestimate the value of hosting sober gatherings. This allows you to control the environment and ensure the focus remains on good old, clean fun. From make-your-own sushi dinner parties and game nights to book clubs or makeover spa nights, you can create engaging experiences that bring people together without substances. Encourage your friends to bring along others who support the sober lifestyle, thus expanding your sober network and strengthening your support system.

REMEMBER

The goal of participating in sober-friendly events and socializ-ing is not just about avoiding substances. It's about enriching your life and creating deeper relationships with like-minded individuals. Focusing on quality interactions and meaningful activities ensures that your sobriety is sustainable and enjoyable in the long run.

Building connections within recovery communities

Whether you are new to sobriety or in long-term recovery, involvement in support groups or sober networks provides a foundation for mutual support and understanding. These con-nections serve as a critical safety net when facing challenges in your sobriety.

BUILDING COMMUNITY WITH JACKSON

My journey into the heart of a recovery community began in silence, almost without me noticing, at a time when I felt utterly disconnected from the world around me. The early days of my sobriety were marked not just by the absence of alcohol but by a void left by the lack of understanding from those I once called *friends*. They couldn't see the scale of my daily battle — the sheer force of will it took to turn away from a life slowly unraveling before me.

The game changed for me nine months into sobriety. I ended up at a local recovery meeting — one I'd attended now and then, more because I thought I should rather than out of any real hope for connection. But on that particular evening, something shifted. I'd always listened to the stories shared in that room, tales of hardship, small wins, and the occasional setback. But that night, I truly heard them. I heard my own fears and aspirations echoed in their voices. The room was charged with an energy of electricity that seemed to vibrate in the air, and no alcohol was involved!

Finding courage within, I shared my story, it was incredible, a total out-of-body experience. My voice was shaky at first, heavy with burdens I wished to forget. But as I spoke, the heaviness began to lift, and a new feeling took over — *a sense of belonging*. The supportive nods and kind words that followed felt like a lifeline to someone quietly drowning.

From that moment, my visits to the recovery group became the foundation for my sober life. I was no longer a lone soul on an unforgiving path; I was part of a collective, a community striving together for a brighter, alcohol-free future.

I began to find my place within this community naturally. I started organizing sober activities, like hikes with breathtaking views and movie nights where laughter was our only indulgence. I became a regular contributor in online forums, sharing encouragement and insights from my journey. I have found that helping others through their recovery process reinforced my own, I love it.

(continued)

(continued)

When the chance came to mentor a newcomer, I didn't hesitate. I saw a reflection of my former self in Beck"s apprehensive gaze. Week by week, I witnessed Beck find his footing, much as I had, and with each step he took toward a stable life, my heart swelled with pride. He is getting sober with me. Wow!

Eventually, I found myself facilitating meetings. It was a role that once would have petrified me, but I embraced it with newfound confidence. Looking out at the faces before me, I saw parts of my journey in theirs — all different stories, all tied together by a shared, steadfast resolve to break free from the clutches of addiction.

My story within the recovery community stands as evidence of the transformative power of connections. It shows that while our paths to sobriety are incredibly personal, they don't have to be walked in isolation. Supported by the framework of recovery groups, the warmth found in shared activities, and the give-and-take of mentorship, each person's recovery can be fortified by the collective strength of many. It's a narrative I, and so many others, continue to walk each day with every step we take in committed sobriety.

Engaging with others who share your experience of striving for sobriety enriches your support network. This engagement can be through regular meetings, shared activities, or online forums, where you can exchange stories, offer advice, and garner encouragement. Establishing these ties fosters a sense of belonging and community, invaluable when moments of confusion, doubt, or vulnerability sneak into your ideas. Being part of a recovery group helps reinforce your commitment to sobriety and empowers you to remain firm in your resolve during tough times. Hosting meetings, organizing sober social events, or mentoring newcomers are just a few ways you can deepen your connections and significantly impact your recovery journey and that of others.

Nurturing healthy friendships that support sobriety

Nurturing healthy friendships that support your sobriety is more than just a pleasant add-on to your recovery journey; it's a critical component of your long-term success. These are the relationships where your choice to live sober is respected and celebrated. By spending time with friends who honor your life choices, you create a positive and reinforcing environment that supports your commitment to sobriety. Life is much easier.

Engaging in substance-free activities together is essential. Whether it's hiking, taking a cooking class, volunteering, playing sports, or attending cultural events, these shared experiences can deepen your bonds and provide a sense of joy and fulfillment that once might have been sought through alcohol or drugs. Such activities not only distract from old triggers but also help you to discover new passions and interests.

REMEMBER

The quality of your friendships is vital, not necessarily the number. Friends who genuinely support your sobriety will take the time to understand your journey. They'll listen without judgment, offer encouragement during challenging times, and celebrate your milestones and achievements. These friends serve as a mirror, reflecting back the strength and determination you might not always see in yourself.

A healthy friendship is a two-way street; your understanding and encouragement will also be invaluable to your friends when they face their own challenges. This mutual exchange nurtures a profound level of trust and intimacy that can be incredibly healing and empowering.

Don't shy away from discussing your needs and boundaries with your friends. Honest communication can prevent misunderstandings and ensure your friends know how best to support you. If you find that some of your old friendships are not conducive to your sobriety, it's okay to seek out new connections that align more closely with your current values and lifestyle.

TIP

Patience is important. Building and nurturing these friendships takes time and effort, and the investment is worth it. The encouragement and support you receive from these relationships will be a cornerstone of your sobriety, helping you to remain focused and motivated — no matter what life throws your way.

As you live in long-term recovery, your network of friends isn't just about avoiding substances. It's about enriching your life and providing a foundation of support that sustains you through the ebbs and flows of life.

Having Fun in Sobriety

Nurturing friendships that actively support your sobriety is crucial. This involves spending time with friends who respect your life choices and engage in substance-free activities. Friends who understand and encourage your journey respect your choices and offer a safety net during challenging times. Activities that are free from substances provide a safe environment that reinforces your decision to stay sober. Whether your friends are in sobriety or not, their understanding and encouragement can provide immense support, keeping you focused and motivated on your path to sustained sobriety.

Developing healthy friendships often requires actively initiating outings and events that align with your sobriety goals. Consider hosting a movie night, hiking, or attending local arts and crafts classes together. It is about finding and immersing yourself in joyful and fulfilling experiences that do not revolve around substances. You should seek out peers who prioritize your recovery in their interactions with you, ensuring that each gathering reinforces your life choices.

Now, let's do a sobriety-supportive scavenger hunt with the following goals:

>> Foster connections with friends who support your sobriety.

>> Create a fun, substance-free environment that encourages teamwork and communication.

>> Explore and enjoy the world around you without the presence of alcohol or drugs.

1. **Overview:**

   Everyone loves scavenger hunts! You can organize this activity with your friends, creating a playful and engaging experience supporting your sobriety commitment. The scavenger hunt will encourage you and your friends to work together, communicate, and enjoy a shared sense of achievement — all within a safe and sober setting.

2. **Preparation:**

   - **Form teams:** Invite friends who support your sobriety and divide into small teams.

   - **Create a list:** Develop a list of items and challenges that can be found or performed within a designated area, such as a park, city center, or neighborhood.

   - **Set boundaries:** Clearly outline the boundaries of the scavenger hunt area, ensuring all locations are safe and substance-free.

   - **Establish rules:** Clarify the rules, including a strict no-alcohol and no-drugs policy and respecting all participants' sobriety.

3. **The scavenger hunt:**

   - **Challenges:** Include a mix of physical items to be collected (e.g., a leaf shaped like a heart) and actions to be performed (e.g., complimenting a stranger, group photo in front of a landmark).

   - **Time limit:** Set a reasonable time limit, such as two hours, for teams to complete the scavenger hunt.

   - **Capture the moment:** Encourage teams to document their finds with photos or videos to share with the group at the end of the hunt.

   - **Creativity counts:** Award bonus points for creative approaches to the challenges.

4. **Post-hunt gathering:**

   - **Meetup:** After the scavenger hunt, gather at a predetermined, substance-free location to share experiences and present the documented finds.

- **Celebrate:** Acknowledge all participants' efforts, celebrate the winning team, and discuss everyone's favorite parts of the activity.

- **Reflect:** Use this time to reflect on the benefits of engaging in sober activities and the support you've all provided each other.

5. **Takeaways:**

   - By the end of the scavenger hunt, you will have strengthened your friendships and built new memories in a fun and active way.

   - You'll have reinforced that enjoyment and camaraderie don't require substances.

   - Based on the positive experiences shared during the scavenger hunt, you'll have opened up opportunities for future substance-free activities and gatherings.

This activity creates an enjoyable day with friends and serves as a reminder of the important role of nurturing healthy friendships in your sobriety journey. By actively initiating and participating in events like this, you cultivate a supportive network that values and respects your life choices. Have fun with it.

Exploring hobbies and activities without substance use

In sobriety, embracing hobbies and activities that don't revolve around substance use is a liberating and enriching experience. This journey is much more than just a way to pass the time; it's an opportunity to discover personal interests that past dependencies might have overshadowed. Whether picking up a brush and finding solace in painting, lacing up your boots for a trek through nature, immersing yourself in the complexities of computer code, or experimenting with new recipes in the kitchen, each activity offers a distinct avenue for self-expression and personal growth. By engaging in these endeavors, you slowly peel back the layers of your identity that were once obscured, rediscovering and reforming your sense of self without the crutch of alcohol or drugs.

You may discover their therapeutic benefits as you venture into these new or perhaps forgotten hobbies. Activities like creative arts can foster a meditative state of mind, alleviate stress, and improve overall mental health. Meanwhile, physical activities such as hiking or sports build physical strength and mental resilience, proving that you can conquer challenges without reliance on substances. Social hobbies, like cooking classes or coding workshops, enhance your skills and expand your social network with individuals who share similar interests but might not necessarily be part of the sober community. This broadens your support system and helps reinforce your sobriety by integrating it into a broader lifestyle context.

REMEMBER

The journey of discovery is ongoing. The hobbies you embrace today may evolve or lead to other interests tomorrow. Keep an open communication channel with yourself, acknowledging when a specific activity resonates with your current state of mind and when it's time to try something new!

Planning sober-friendly entertainment and events

Sobriety breathes new life into your social calendar at any length of sobriety, offering a chance to experience genuine enjoyment without the need for alcohol. Embrace your role as a creative planner to curate events and activities that resonate with a sober lifestyle. From cozy movie nights at home to attending live sports, from engaging book discussions to interactive dinner parties, the emphasis is on the richness of the experience, not the presence of alcohol.

Dive into the world of hobbies that keep spirits high without the spirits. Group activities such as bowling, arts and crafts, DIY pizza parties, or outdoor fitness classes become more than just pastimes; they are opportunities to connect and form bonds with others who appreciate your commitment to a sober life. When planning these gatherings, prioritize inclusivity and comfort, creating an environment where the joy of togetherness is the main attraction.

Cultural outings, like theater shows, live music, and art galleries, add variety and depth to your entertainment options, often in settings less focused on alcohol. Organize outings with sober friends or identify sober sections at these events to maintain a supportive network and enjoy public spaces confidently.

TIP

Keep a "sober plan B" handy for when social plans unexpectedly change or if you find yourself in a situation where alcohol is present. This could be as simple as having a list of local cafes that offer live music, knowing the schedule for the nearby art gallery, or carrying the details for a spontaneous evening walk or movie night. Having alternatives at the ready allows you to take control of your social life and maintain your sobriety with confidence. Remember, it's not just about avoiding alcohol — it's about crafting fulfilling experiences that support your lifestyle.

Taking on the role of host can transform your living space into a bastion of sobriety, where non-alcoholic cookouts, board game marathons, or private film festivals celebrate connection without the need for intoxication. Tailor the atmosphere to be welcoming and secure, showcasing a range of delicious non-alcoholic options and fostering genuine interactions.

Your proactive approach to designing and enjoying sober-friendly events reinforces your dedication to a sober lifestyle. It also invites others to recognize the rich, vibrant reality of life in recovery.

REMEMBER

Your commitment to sobriety doesn't mean you have to sacrifice a vibrant social life. It's about reshaping your entertainment to fit your new lifestyle. Always take the time to communicate your plans and boundaries with your social circle, and never hesitate to assert your needs. Embrace your role as a planner with the knowledge that you're crafting a social life that's safe and supportive of your sobriety and deeply rewarding.

Chapter **15**

Developing Coping Mechanisms and Resilience (Mindfulness)

I magine a blank notebook, ready for you to fill its pages. You are the writer, and your tools are mindfulness and sobriety. Each entry represents a moment of presence, a decision to engage with life authentically, free from the haze of alcohol or a harsh judging mind. The beauty of this work lies not in its perfection but in its unique journey — a journey of resilience, clarity, and profound transformation.

In this chapter, you will embark on a journey through the world of present-moment awareness. Mindfulness is a gentle anchor in the now, which steers you from the tumultuous waves of past and future worries. It is a compassionate guide, teaching you to embrace each experience with equanimity and grace. You'll discover how the simple act of being fully engaged in the here and now can illuminate the path to sobriety, fortifying your resolve against life's ebbs and flows. As you unfold the pages of this chapter, you'll find practical tools and mindful exercises that weave tranquility into the fabric of your daily life, strengthening your resilience with every mindful breath.

Introduction to Mindfulness Practices

Understanding that mindfulness can be a foundational practice within your recovery is essential. Mindfulness is the deliberate act of attentively engaging with the here and now while peacefully recognizing and accepting one's emotions, thoughts, and physical sensations. It's a therapeutic technique rooted in meditation but applicable in everyday life. Mindfulness can be a powerful ally in your recovery, complementing the strategies outlined in previous chapters. For example, when you are eating a balanced meal as described in Chapter 8, you are engaged in mindful eating. This means you choose nutritious foods and take time to *experience* eating with all your senses.

Incorporating mindfulness techniques can enrich the practices for maintaining sobriety outlined in the "Nature Versus Nurture in Family Relations" chapter found on www.dummies.com. If your routine includes a morning run, use this time to practice mindfulness by fully experiencing the rhythm of your stride, the pattern of your breath, and the changing environment around you.

TIP

To access the online chapter mentioned in this section and other helpful sobriety materials, visit www.dummies.com and search for this book's title.

The advantages of integrating mindfulness into your recovery process are significant and far-reaching. Besides reducing stress and improving emotional regulation, which is beneficial for everyone, mindfulness explicitly helps those in recovery by providing tools to manage cravings and emotional discomfort.

Mindfulness encourages you to observe these experiences without judgment and to understand that they are transient, giving you the strength to make choices that support your sobriety.

Mindfulness transcends a mere practice; it is a lifestyle that can profoundly augment your journey to sustained long-term recovery. It supports the serenity and clarity you've worked to foster throughout your journey. Integrating mindfulness into your daily routine and embracing it as a regular part of your life sets the stage for a richer, more connected, sober experience.

TIP

To ground your recovery in mindfulness, begin by dedicating a moment to fully engage with a single task each day. Whether it's mindful eating by savoring every bite of your meal or engaging all your senses during a morning walk, make it a point to immerse yourself completely in the experience. This conscious effort to be present can dramatically shift your relationship with daily activities, turning them from routine to enriching moments that support your sobriety. Start small with one activity, and gradually expand this mindful approach to other aspects of your life for a more centered and fulfilling recovery journey.

Mindfulness versus mindlessness

Embarking on the topic of mindfulness versus mindlessness invites you to consider the quality of your daily experiences. Imagine the vibrancy of your life when you are living in high definition — the sharpness of colors, the clarity of sounds, and the depth of sensations. Mindfulness offers you this heightened sense of living, where every moment is an opportunity for full participation and appreciation. This vivid awareness contrasts sharply with the foggy haze of mindlessness, where life's intricate details are lost to a disconnected and automatic existence. You would live on *autopilot*, not sensing, just robotically moving about your day, with nothing changing. You could also associate this way of living with the onset of complacency, where and when a spark can occur, and place your recovery in danger. As you navigate your recovery, the choice between mindfulness and mindlessness can shape the texture of your days — will you choose the vividness of the present or the obscurity of disengagement?

Pause for a moment to explore the distinctions between a mindful and mindless existence with this guided exercise:

1. Seek out a peaceful environment where you can sit undisturbed and at ease.

2. Engage in three deliberate, deep inhalations and exhalations, directing your full attention to the path the breath takes through your body.

3. Contemplate a habitual activity you perform daily, such as tooth brushing. Reflect on your normal conduct during this task.

4. Pose the following inquiries to yourself:

   - During tooth brushing, is my mind often elsewhere, perhaps planning the day ahead or revisiting past events?

   - Am I attuned to the sensation of the toothbrush bristles dancing along my gumline, the flavor profile of the toothpaste, and the invigorating cleanness permeating my mouth afterward?

   If your answers align more with the first question, you may tend toward mindlessness. However, if you resonate with the second, it may indicate a mindfulness practice. This simple exercise can serve as a mirror, revealing instances where your presence wanes, and in turn, it can guide you to infuse your everyday tasks with greater presence and mindfulness.

REMEMBER

Mindfulness is about engaging fully with the present, even in routine activities. Notice whether your mind wanders during tasks like tooth brushing or if you're truly sensing the experience. A mindful approach to everyday actions increases your awareness and enhances your recovery by fostering a deeper connection with the present moment. Keep this distinction in mind to prevent slipping into mindlessness and reinforce the habits supporting your sobriety and well-being.

Incorporating mindfulness into your daily routine can seem challenging, especially if you are used to a lifestyle marked by constant activity and distraction. Yet, the benefits of this practice are profound, including reduced stress, improved emotional regulation, and enhanced self-awareness. Mindfulness exercises, such as deep breathing, guided imagery, or even simple attentive listening, can be practical tools to bring you back to the present moment. These techniques foster a sense of calm and control, essential for managing cravings and dealing with life's unpredictabilities.

Mindfulness can strengthen your ability to handle emotional discomfort without resorting to old habits of substance abuse or other negative coping strategies. Mindfulness empowers you to choose responses that align with your long-term goals and values by teaching you to sit with uncomfortable feelings and understand their transient nature. The integrated mindfulness approach supports your sobriety and enhances overall life satisfaction and connectedness. Embracing these practices as a regular part of your life will undoubtedly pave the way for a richer, more fulfilling, sober journey.

TIP

To integrate mindfulness seamlessly into your busy life, start with simple, brief exercises that reset your focus to the present. Try scheduling short breaks for deep breathing or mindful observation throughout your day. This can be as easy as pausing to listen intently to the sounds around you or taking a moment to consciously relax your muscles. These practices can quickly become second nature, helping you maintain tranquility, navigate emotional challenges, and reinforce your commitment to sobriety with each mindful act.

Understanding the basics of mindfulness

As elucidated by Dr. Judson Brewer, psychiatrist and neuroscientist, and supported by robust neuroscientific evidence, mindfulness is the *practice* of maintaining a moment-by-moment awareness of your thoughts, emotions, bodily sensations, and surrounding environment with openness and curiosity. It involves a kind of attentiveness to the present that notices without clinging to or rejecting what is noticed, fostering a sense of presence that is both grounding and liberating.

Dr. Brewer's work has shed light on what happens in the brain during mindfulness practice, particularly with respect to addiction. His research indicates that mindfulness can modulate the activity of the prefrontal cortex — the area of the brain responsible for self-regulation and executive function. This modulation can weaken the grip of craving-related circuits, diminishing the pull of habit patterns associated with addiction. Mindfulness training has been shown to increase the density of gray matter in the prefrontal cortex, enhancing your capacity to control automatic impulses.

It's also been discovered that mindfulness can alter the functioning of the default mode network (DMN), which is active when the mind is wandering and not focused on the outside world, often involved in self-referential thoughts, including those related to craving and addiction. Through practicing mindfulness, you can learn to observe these patterns of mind wandering and craving with a detached curiosity, which, in effect, disempowers them.

TIP

You can leverage the power of mindfulness to transform your brain and combat addiction by starting with a simple yet profound practice: focused breathing. Dedicate a few minutes each day to sit quietly and concentrate solely on your breath. Inhale slowly, observing the sensation of the air entering your nostrils, filling your lungs, and expanding your chest and belly. Then, exhale gently, noticing the release of tension and the following natural relaxation. This practice can enhance the neural pathways in your prefrontal cortex, aiding you in managing impulses and cravings with greater ease. As you cultivate this habit, you'll begin to witness a decrease in the mind's tendency to wander and a stronger, more self-regulated response to the *sparks* of addiction.

Habit loops

Incorporating the insights drawn from the work of Judson Brewer and understanding that your brain is addicted to certain habits, let's consider a tool he came to as habit mapping. This tool is paramount when addressing addiction recovery. This tool is a practical framework for deconstructing the cycles that underpin addictive behaviors. His model focuses on identifying the elements of the habit loop (see Figure 15-1): the cue, the behavior, and the reward.

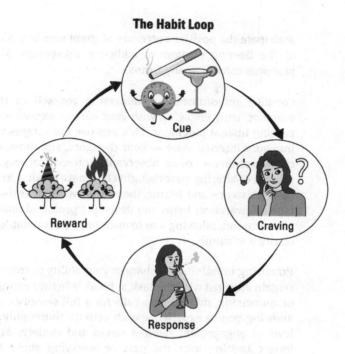

The Habit Loop

Cue

Craving

Response

Reward

FIGURE 15-1:
Habit loops.

In the context of your recovery journey, mapping out your habit loops can be transformative. The cue triggers your behavior; the signal ignites the automatic urge to engage in the addictive action. The behavior is the action you take in response to the cue, and the reward is the outcome that your brain learns to associate with that behavior, perpetuating the cycle.

Understanding this loop provides a strategic advantage in recovery, as it allows you to intercept the process and implement alternative actions. When you notice the cue — perhaps a stressful moment or a certain time of day — you can choose a behavior that aligns with your recovery goals. This could be reaching out to a support network, engaging in deep breathing exercises, or immersing yourself in a distraction that offers fulfillment without the detrimental consequences of substance use.

You begin to rewrite your habit loops as you repeatedly choose these healthier behaviors and experience the rewards — such as a sense of control, improved well-being, or simply the pride of sticking to your sobriety. This process *does not happen overnight*, but with consistent effort and mindfulness, your brain learns to anticipate the positive outcomes of these new behaviors instead of the fleeting comfort of addictive substances. Mindfulness practices come in many forms.

Consider mindfulness as immersing yourself in the present moment, truly engaging with your current experiences without passing instant judgment. This practice encourages you to tune into your internal state — your thoughts, emotions, and physical sensations — in an observant, non-critical way. It's not a process of altering your thoughts but more about acknowledging their existence and letting them exist without resistance. This type of awareness helps you develop a profound understanding of your mind, allowing you to encounter daily complexities with clarity and calm.

Practicing mindfulness enhances your ability to concentrate and remain engaged with the task at hand. Whether eating, walking, or conversing, mindfulness calls for a full sensory engagement, allowing you to experience each activity thoroughly. This deep level of engagement reduces stress and anxiety, as you're no longer fretting over the past or worrying about the future. Instead, you're giving your full attention to the now, which is inherently calming and can significantly boost your overall mental health.

The role of mindfulness in coping mechanisms

Mindfulness equips you with the ability to confront rather than avoid the emotional turbulence often encountered in recovery. As you develop mindfulness, you learn that resilience isn't just about enduring hardship and growing from experiences without reverting to old, destructive habits. This readiness to face life's ups and downs head-on is a crucial coping mechanism that sustains long-term sobriety and personal growth.

Understanding and developing coping mechanisms is vital. Coping mechanisms are automatic psychological processes that help you manage stress, emotions, and thoughts that could lead to relapse. Mindfulness enhances these mechanisms by fostering a non-reactive awareness of the present moment, allowing you to notice and acknowledge cravings, stressors, or sparks without being overwhelmed by them.

Why is this important for you in recovery? Because the very nature of addiction involves a loss of control over behaviors in response to stimuli. During active addiction, coping mechanisms often involve substance use to manage uncomfortable emotions or situations. In recovery, however, it's about replacing those destructive patterns with healthy, life-affirming ones.

Mindfulness practices, which reference Jon Kabat-Zinn's scientifically backed mindfulness-based stress reduction (MBSR) techniques, can be instrumental in rewiring the brain. These practices help strengthen the prefrontal cortex — the part of your brain involved in decision-making and impulse control. Enhancing its function gives you more control over your responses to cravings.

TIP

Mindfulness can be a cornerstone in your recovery, offering a way to directly experience the present moment without the automatic reactions that often can lead to relapse. To integrate mindfulness, start by dedicating time each day to simply notice your thoughts, sensations, and feelings without judgment. Remember, it's about progress, not perfection; each mindful moment is a step toward sustainable recovery.

Neuroscientific studies, like those mentioned in Chapter 8 and found in the resources from the National Institute on Alcohol Abuse and Alcoholism and PubMed Central, show that mindfulness affects the DMN related to self-referential thoughts and mind wandering. A hyperactive DMN is often associated with cravings and addiction. Mindfulness can modulate this activity, allowing you to become an observer of your thoughts rather than a participant in them.

The research highlighted in Chapter 3 emphasizes that mindfulness can help you develop emotional regulation — managing how you experience and respond to emotions. This is crucial, as your sobriety journey often involves navigating intense emotional landscapes.

In essence, mindfulness is a foundational practice supporting all other coping mechanisms. It encourages growth from within, allowing you to confront and grow from experiences without the need for substance use. It's about nurturing a strong, resilient self that can face life's myriad challenges with clarity and calm.

REMEMBER

Recovery is not just about abstaining from substances; it's about building a life that you don't want to escape from. Mindfulness is a key tool in that construction, offering a way to live in alignment with your goals, values, and the essence of who you are beyond addiction.

Benefits of incorporating mindfulness in recovery

Integrating mindfulness into your recovery process has scientifically proven benefits that extend to neurological aspects of your health. Studies indicate that regular mindfulness practices can reshape the patterns in your brain connected to stress, anxiety, and craving. These changes are significant because they enhance your cognitive abilities and stabilize your emotional responses, thereby supporting your journey toward sobriety and improved overall health.

Scientific studies reveal the following:

» **Enhanced cognitive control**

Mindfulness has been shown to strengthen the prefrontal cortex, the area of the brain responsible for decision-making, focus, and impulse control. This can help you resist the urge to relapse and make choices that support your sobriety.

» **Regulation of the stress response**

The amygdala, which is involved in processing stress and fear, becomes less reactive through mindfulness. This can lessen anxiety and the body's stress response, which can be triggers for substance use.

>> **Improved emotional regulation**

With regular practice, mindfulness can alter the function of the DMN, which is active during mind-wandering and self-referential thoughts — a state often linked to depression and anxiety. Training the mind to remain present can help decrease ruminative thinking patterns that might lead to relapse.

>> **Neuroplasticity**

Mindfulness promotes neuroplasticity, the brain's ability to form new neural connections throughout life. This means that the more you engage in mindfulness practices, the more you reinforce the neural pathways that help you manage cravings and respond healthily to stress.

>> **Decreased craving response**

Mindfulness can change your relationship with cravings. By observing cravings without judgment, you can learn to ride them out without acting on them, reducing their intensity over time.

>> **Altered reward processing**

Addiction can hijack the brain's reward system, but mindfulness meditation has been shown to modulate the activity in brain regions associated with the reward circuitry, potentially resetting your brain's reward system to find pleasure in non-substance-related activities.

Scientific underpinnings of mindfulness in recovery highlight that this practice can lead to tangible changes in brain function and structure, which support long-term sobriety. These benefits go beyond managing your addiction; they extend to enhancing your overall mental health and well-being.

REMEMBER

It's essential to approach mindfulness practice consistently to gain these benefits, and it's always a good idea to seek guidance from a trained professional, especially when integrating it into a recovery program. Mindfulness can complement other treatment modalities, making it a versatile tool in the quest for sustained sobriety.

THE UNFOLDING OF A MINDFUL RECOVERY WITH DUNCAN

Perched at my desk with a view of the city's constant motion, I was starkly aware of a gnawing discomfort inside me. Despite a decade of sobriety and all the outward signs of a life well-built, I was wrestling with an irritability that clung to my every day. True contentment, a deep sense of peace, and a zest for living every day was elusive. It was as if it hung in the night sky — visible yet out of reach. My dedication to the 12-step program was solid, yet the promise of inner calm seemed to taunt me. I was becoming more and more unhappy.

I was in a state of inner turmoil when mindfulness entered my life. Seeing my silent struggle, a friend suggested mindfulness as a lifeline. "There's science behind it," he insisted, appealing to my logical nature. I was hesitant, but the relentless internal clamor pushed me to try anything that promised even a whisper of relief.

I started with meditation — once a day, every day — immersing myself in staying rooted in the present. It wasn't easy, but I kept at it. The early days were a battle against my own mind's wanderings; I was determined. I remembered reading about the resilience that comes from mindfulness in a newspaper posting months before trying it.

Gradually, my thoughts began to change, and the negativity that always seemed to be present started to shift. My cravings that once hung around like looming specters became more like passing clouds — observable but not overpowering. Stressful office moments, once my doing, were now met with a surprising calm. It was as if the mindfulness was rewiring my brain, strengthening my thinking for better decision-making and emotional regulation.

My evolution was not only internal. Others noticed a newfound poise in my interactions — my thoughts were clearer, and my reflexes to life's provocations were more measured. This new version of me — collected, conscious, *present* — was a product of the new pathways etched into my brain by my dedication to mindfulness.

As the months and years passed, my commitment to this practice did not waver. The simple act of breathing with intention brought me a serenity that my ten-year sobriety chip alone had not. I realized that while external achievements brought fleeting happiness, this internal cultivation of mindfulness offered me sustainable joy. I realized that while external achievements brought fleeting happiness, this internal cultivation of mindfulness offered me sustainable joy.

Now, when I share my story, I do so not just as a government official or an individual in long-term recovery but as a man who found contentment through the deliberate practice of mindfulness. My life, once at the mercy of an addiction narrative, now gently unfolds in a calm rhythm, a daily testament to the quiet yet profound strength of my mindful existence.

Mindfulness Techniques for Coping with Stress

You can learn to cope with stress healthily and effectively by embracing mindfulness techniques. These practices help you stay centered and respond to life's challenges with more composure and less impulsivity.

One fundamental technique is focused breathing, which calms the mind and steadies emotions. When you feel overwhelmed, taking deep, structured breaths can shift your mental state, providing immediate relief from acute stress. This exercise helps manage stress in the moment and trains your brain to remain calm under pressure over time.

Here are additional techniques:

» Body scan meditation

Lie down and mentally scan your body from head to toe, noticing any areas of tension and consciously relaxing them.

» Walking meditation

Take a leisurely walk and pay attention to the sensation of your feet touching the ground, the rhythm of your steps, and the movement of your body.

» Guided imagery

Visualize a peaceful scene, such as a beach or a forest. Engage all your senses to immerse yourself fully in this place of calm.

» Mindful observation

Choose an object around you and focus all your attention on it. Observe the details, texture, and colors, allowing your mind to become absorbed in the process.

» Mindful eating

Eat slowly and savor each bite, paying attention to your food's flavors, textures, and aromas.

» Compassion meditation

Send thoughts of love and kindness to yourself and others. This practice can create a sense of connectedness and reduce feelings of isolation.

» Progressive muscle relaxation

Tense and then relax each muscle group, starting with your toes and working your way up to your head. This can help release physical and mental tension.

» Journaling

Take time daily to reflect and write down your thoughts. This can help you become more aware of internal stressors and patterns in your thinking.

» Mindfulness bell

Set a reminder on your phone or use an app to sound a bell at random intervals. Each time you hear the bell, pause and take a moment to breathe and center yourself.

REMEMBER

The key is to practice these techniques regularly and with intention. They may seem simple, but they have a profound effect on your ability to manage stress and maintain your sobriety. Each technique can be a stepping stone to greater resilience and emotional stability.

An intersection of two practices — mindfulness and stoicism

Stoicism, a philosophy with ancient roots, provides a robust framework for personal development, especially when combined with mindfulness, a cornerstone of mental well-being. Stoicism teaches the art of living virtuously and with emotional intelligence by focusing on what's within your control while accepting what you cannot change. It emphasizes rational thinking, personal accountability, and the importance of aligning your actions with your values.

The stoic practice of premeditation malorum — the premeditation of adversities — involves anticipating potential challenges and preparing oneself to face them with *equanimity*. This mental rehearsal aligns closely with mindfulness, encouraging a non-reactive awareness of thoughts and feelings as they arise. By integrating stoic foresight with the attentive calm of mindfulness, individuals in recovery can navigate the uncertainties of life and interpersonal relationships with greater composure and less distress.

When stoicism and mindfulness are woven together, they form a practical toolkit for living in sobriety. Both approaches teach you to engage with the present moment without judgment. This dual practice fosters resilience, reduces stress, and bolsters your ability to remain sober, even when faced with life's inevitable challenges.

TIP

Each morning, take a moment to visualize the day ahead. Consider potential challenges and remind yourself that while you can't control every circumstance, you have power over your reactions. Pair this stoic exercise with a brief mindfulness meditation, observing your thoughts and emotions and creating a calm inner environment. This prepares you to face the day with a balanced and intentional mindset, reinforcing your commitment to recovery.

Mindful stoic relations

In the recovery journey, relationships often serve as both cornerstone and crucible, offering support and sometimes presenting challenges that test the resilience you've built in your sober life. The practices of stoicism and mindfulness provide invaluable tools for navigating the social sphere with deliberate intention and emotional composure.

Stoicism reminds you that not every action of others is within your control, but your responses are. When a friend cancels plans or a family member brings up a sensitive topic, stoicism teaches you to respond rather than react, preserving inner peace by focusing on what's within your control — your perceptions, decisions, and behaviors.

Mindfulness complements this by encouraging an open, non-judgmental awareness of the present moment. It allows you to recognize your emotional reactions to interpersonal dynamics without becoming overwhelmed by them. When you're mindful, you're better equipped to communicate effectively, listen actively, and build deeper connections.

You can employ these practices in your relationships, engaging with kindness and assertiveness, setting healthy boundaries, and approaching conflicts with a clear, calm mind. For instance, if a disagreement arises, stoicism can help you stay aligned with your core values, while mindfulness can keep you rooted in the present, reducing the likelihood of being swept away by anger or resentment.

By living with these principles of stoicism and mindfulness, you create routines that support and enhance your interactions. You learn to cultivate nurturing and resilient relationships that can weather the storms of recovery and heal the wounds of the past.

For further exploration, consider revisiting the chapters on fostering resilience (as discussed in Chapter 3).

EXPECT THE EXPECTED AND LEARN TO LOVE IT WITH DEREK

Often, we are told in life that we should expect the unexpected. To be ready for those moments in life when something happens or someone behaves in a way we could never possibly imagine. It can seem helpful to live life with this way of thinking so that we are always prepared for those surprises that can throw our lives out of balance.

But is this the best advice for handling others?

Stoic philosophers believe we should always expect the expected when it comes to other people. If we can mentally prepare ourselves for what a person might say or how they might act in a given situation, then when things play out the way that we predicted, we should have a better chance of defusing situations and avoiding conflicts.

Think of someone you might struggle with personally — someone who says or does things that get under your skin. It could be a family member, coworker, or neighbor. Think about what they might say or things that they might do that bother you. If you have been around this person enough, then you should be able to easily figure out what that might be.

Now, when you are about to have an interaction with this person again, take a moment to tell yourself what you should expect. Predict what they might say to you and what actions they might take. And when things happen how you predicted, then you should not be surprised. After all, did you expect anything different based on how it normally goes with them?

My mother will go out of her way to embarrass me. I think she takes personal pride in doing that. She tells complete strangers in public about my childhood and my later addictions. I have told her how it bothers me, but she continues to do it. So, when I am going to be around her now, I tell myself that I expect her to go out of her way to reveal things about me to utter strangers. And when she does this, just as I predicted, I am less bothered because I had expected it.

(continued)

(continued)

> You cannot avoid all interpersonal conflicts in life, but you have to ask yourself how many conflicts occur with people who do and say things they always do and say. Expecting anything different from them would not make sense. Try to live your life by expecting the expected when it comes to other people, helping you decrease the number of conflicts.

The stoic circle of influence in relationships

This exercise draws upon the stoic principle we've been sharing differentiating between what is within your control and what is not, helping you cultivate more meaningful and less reactive relationships in your recovery journey. You'll need your favorite pen and paper or a digital note-taking device and find a quiet space for reflection.

Follow these instructions:

>> **Identify relationships that you want to work on:** List the significant relationships in your life, including family, friends, colleagues, and acquaintances.

>> **Assess influence:** Next to each name, note whether their actions are within your control, influence, or entirely outside your control.

>> **Determine responses:** Reflect on recent interactions with each person. Write down instances where you reacted to something outside of your control and consider how you could respond more stoically next time.

>> **Envision scenarios:** Visualize potential future scenarios with these individuals. Imagine them acting in a way that challenges you, and practice framing your response with stoic calmness, focusing on what you can control — your own actions and attitude.

>> **Practice mindful awareness:** Incorporate mindfulness by becoming aware of your immediate emotional responses in these visualizations. Acknowledge your feelings without

judgment and then guide your focus back to your stoic response.

>> **Commit to daily practice:** Commit to practicing this stoic mindfulness in real-time interactions, taking a deep breath before responding to any situation, and reminding yourself of your circle of influence.

>> **Reflect and adjust:** At the end of each day, reflect on your interactions. Celebrate when you successfully maintained composure and learn from the times you did not.

By consistently applying this exercise, you reinforce the *stoic mindset* in your relationships, leading to more harmonious interactions and a supportive environment conducive to long-term recovery.

REMEMBER

As discussed earlier in this chapter, developing coping mechanisms through mindfulness is not just about avoidance; it's about actively engaging in your recovery by choosing responses that align with your values and goals.

MBSR in long-term recovery

MBSR is a clinically proven program designed to alleviate stress, pain, and illness by integrating mindful awareness into your daily life. Developed by Dr. Jon Kabat-Zinn at the University of Massachusetts Medical School, MBSR teaches mindfulness meditation and gentle yoga to cultivate awareness and reduce stress.

MBSR's effectiveness lies in its structured approach to nurturing mindfulness — a kind of mental state marked by nonjudgmental awareness of the present moment. Mindfulness techniques focus on breath, bodily sensations, and mental content while acknowledging and accepting feelings, thoughts, and bodily sensations.

In the realm of addiction recovery, MBSR's significance cannot be overstated. Joseph Goldstein, a notable mindfulness teacher, emphasizes that mindfulness training can significantly improve your capacity to manage stress and emotions — key factors often contributing to relapse. MBSR helps break the automatic and habitual reactions that can lead to inner turmoil, enabling you to be more reflective instead of reflexive to stressors.

By engaging in structured meditation as part of MBSR, you can develop a deepened awareness of the present moment, minimizing distractions and enhancing your concentration. This practice involves focusing on your breath or a particular object, making you more attuned to your body's responses to stress and anxiety. Over time, this leads to greater emotional regulation and a calm mind, even in challenging situations.

Neuroscientific research supports the use of mindfulness in recovery. Structural changes in the brain associated with increased gray matter concentration in areas related to learning, memory, emotion regulation, self-referential processing, and perspective-taking have been documented in individuals practicing mindfulness meditation. These brain changes are especially beneficial for you as you continue your sobriety, as they enhance your ability to regulate emotions and cope with the cravings and sparks often encountered during your long-term sobriety journey.

Clinical studies have demonstrated that patients who undergo MBSR training can experience a reduction in the use of substances as well as significant decreases in levels of stress and emotional distress. The MBSR program is quite effective in supporting those with emotional dysregulation.

For individuals in long-term recovery, MBSR offers a scientifically backed, non-pharmacological approach to maintaining sobriety and enhancing overall well-being. By improving emotional intelligence, fostering resilience, and reducing stress, MBSR equips you with the tools to navigate recovery challenges with greater composure and stability.

Integrating MBSR into your routine can be a transformative step in your recovery process. It is a practical investment in your health — both mental and physical — that resonates with the lifelong commitment you've made to your sobriety.

The holistic nature of MBSR encourages a comprehensive lifestyle adjustment toward mindfulness. It's about more than just temporary relief; it's about cultivating a sustained, mindful approach to life. You are learning to relieve stress and perceive life's challenges less reactively and more responsively. This continuous practice ensures that mindfulness becomes a foundational aspect of your life, improving overall well-being.

A step-by-step guide to practicing MBSR

MBSR is a structured program that aims to enhance mindfulness through practiced awareness and acceptance of one's moment-to-moment experience. It is particularly beneficial for individuals in long-term recovery from alcoholism and addiction, as it fosters emotional regulation, stress reduction, and increased well-being.

1. An introduction to mindfulness meditation:

- **Begin with education:** Learn what mindfulness is and how it can support your recovery. Joseph Goldstein, a renowned mindfulness teacher, provides insights into mindfulness as a nonjudgmental, present-moment awareness. The foundational principles of MBSR, developed by Dr. Jon Kabat-Zinn, emphasize mindfulness as a key tool for managing stress and emotions and reducing the likelihood of relapse.

- **Practice mindful breathing:** Sit in a quiet space, close your eyes, and focus on your breath. Notice the sensation of air entering and leaving your body. When your mind wanders, gently bring your focus back to your breath.

- **Try body scan meditation:** Lie down in a comfortable position. Starting from your toes and moving upward, bring your attention to each part of your body. Notice any tension, pain, or discomfort without judgment and breathe into these sensations.

2. Incorporating yoga or gentle stretching:

- **Practice simple yoga:** Engage in gentle, mindful yoga to connect with your body. Focus on each movement and notice how your body feels during the stretches without pushing beyond your comfort level.

- **Walk mindfully:** Take a slow walk, paying close attention to the physical sensations in your legs and feet with each step and the sounds and sights around you.

3. **Daily mindfulness exercises:**

   - **Set routine activities:** Choose daily activities, such as showering or getting into your car when leaving the house. Practice performing each activity with full attention to every detail.

   - **Eat mindfully:** During meals, focus fully on the experience of eating and not doing anything else; no phone, text, books, and so on. Pay attention to your food's colors, textures, flavors, and aromas.

4. **Mindfulness to navigate recovery challenges:**

   - **Recognize your sparks:** Use mindfulness to recognize and manage sparks in your environment. Observe the feelings and thoughts that arise without acting on them impulsively.

   - **Cope with cravings:** When cravings occur, practice mindfulness to observe them as temporary states that will pass. Focus on your breath and bodily sensations to ground yourself in the present.

5. **Integrate MBSR into your daily life:**

   - **Practice regularly:** Dedicate a specific time each day for mindfulness practice, whether it's meditation, yoga, or mindful walking.

   - **Mindfully interact:** Before engaging in conversations or meetings, take a few mindful breaths, pause and center yourself, and be fully present.

   - **Practice mindful reflection:** End each day with a reflection on moments where you were fully present and areas where you can improve.

6. **Additional support:**

   - **Try group sessions or MBSR courses:** Consider joining an MBSR course or group to deepen your practice and connect with others.

   - **Use technology aids:** Use apps or recordings by mindfulness experts like Joseph Goldstein to guide your practice.

7. **Understand mindfulness and the brain:**

- Neuroscience shows that MBSR can lead to structural changes in the brain associated with reduced stress and improved emotional regulation, important factors in maintaining long-term recovery.

REMEMBER

Following these steps and incorporating MBSR into your life can foster the mental resilience necessary for long-term recovery. Mindfulness is a skill that strengthens with practice, and it's okay to start small and build over time. Each mindful moment contributes to a solid foundation of sobriety and health.

Mindfulness Techniques

There are many techniques to discover. What works for one person may not work for you. Explore these practical techniques that can help you manage stress and enhance your well-being during your recovery journey. Mindful breathing to relaxation exercises, these techniques are designed to be integrated into your daily life, offering you powerful tools to maintain balance and foster resilience. Some essential techniques are explained in the following sections.

Mindful breathing and relaxation exercises

Mindful breathing and relaxation exercises are foundational tools you can implement immediately to enhance your emotional and physical well-being. These practices encourage you to focus on your breath, facilitating a grounding experience that reduces any anxiety or stress you may be experiencing. Integrating daily deep, controlled breathing sessions creates a calm space in your mind, allowing for more apparent thoughts and improved stress management.

Starting your day with mindful breathing can set a positive tone for the hours ahead. When you begin with just a few minutes of deep breathing, you actively lower your body's stress response, which can lead to a more composed and mindful approach to your day. This practice doesn't require any special equipment or environment and can be done anywhere you feel comfortable. Consistency is key; turning this into a regular practice can significantly enhance its benefits.

In addition to mindful breathing, relaxation exercises such as progressive muscle relaxation or guided imagery further help in managing stress and anxiety. In progressive muscle relaxation, you systematically tense and then relax different muscle groups, which can effectively release physical tension and promote a sense of physical and mental relaxation. Guided imagery involves visualizing a calm, peaceful setting and engaging all your senses to enhance the feeling of tranquility. This technique aids in reducing stress and also helps improve your overall mood and state of well-being.

Incorporating these practices into your daily, weekly, and monthly routine, especially during high stress or anxiety, can prove invaluable. As you create a personal toolbox of techniques, you will draw upon each to maintain balance and stay grounded. Regularly dedicating time to these exercises strengthens your ability to focus and remain present.

Mindful observation of thoughts and emotions

Observing your thoughts and emotions without judgment is a powerful tool in mindfulness practice that can significantly enhance your ability to cope with daily challenges. This technique encourages you to simply notice your feelings and thoughts as they come without attaching labels or value judgments. By doing so, you can better understand the patterns and triggers of your mental landscape, promoting a more transparent, more objective view of your inner experiences. Gradually, this practice helps reduce the overwhelming influence of negative emotions and thoughts on your overall well-being.

The key to mindful observation is to watch your thoughts as an impartial spectator. Imagine each thought and emotion as a leaf floating down a stream; they arrive, are there for a moment, and then continue down the stream. This mental imagery reinforces the idea that your thoughts and emotions are transient and not an intrinsic part of your identity. Over time, you will find it easier to detach from troubling thoughts and panic-inducing emotions, fostering a calmer and more centered mental state.

As your practice deepens, you might notice a shift in how you react to stressful situations or emotional challenges. This is because mindful observation equips you to recognize and pause automatic responses to stimuli, allowing you to choose how to act or think in a given situation. By integrating mindful observation into your daily routine, you not only enhance your emotional self-regulation but also open up new pathways to personal growth and resilience.

The stream of consciousness — mindful observation

In this exercise, you will practice observing your thoughts and emotions as they arise, without judgment, just as you would watch leaves floating down a stream. This technique helps you become more acquainted with your mental patterns and gain greater control over your responses to them.

You will need a quiet, comfortable space and time. Follow these instructions:

1. Settle in:

- Find a comfortable seated position in a quiet space where you won't be disturbed.

- Set your timer for a reasonable amount of time to start, perhaps 5-10 minutes.

2. Use focused relaxation:

- Close your eyes and take several deep breaths, focusing on the sensation of the air moving in and out of your lungs.

- With each exhale, allow your body to release any tension.

3. **Practice stream visualization:**

   - Visualize a gentle stream in your mind's eye. Envision the water flowing smoothly, surrounded by the serenity of nature.

4. **Observe thoughts and emotions:**

   - As thoughts or emotions bubble up, visualize them as leaves that have fallen into the stream.

   - See each thought or emotion as a leaf floating on the water's surface, being carried away by the current.

   - Avoid grabbing onto the leaves or judging them; simply observe them as they drift by.

5. **Return to your breathing:**

   - Whenever you get swept away by a thought or emotion (grabbing a leaf), gently bring your attention back to the visual of the leaves floating on the water.

   - Re-anchor yourself in the moment by focusing on your breath.

6. **Conclude the exercise:**

   - When your timer goes off, slowly bring your awareness back to the room.

   - Wiggle your fingers and toes and gently open your eyes.

   - Reflect on the experience, acknowledging the various thoughts and emotions that passed through without criticism or attachment.

7. **Practice regularly:**

   - Practice this exercise daily. As you become more comfortable, you can extend the duration of the exercise.

8. **Reflective integration:**

   - After completing the exercise, consider jotting down any insights or patterns you observed. Did certain types of thoughts or emotions appear more frequently? Did you notice any shift in how you relate to them? By documenting these observations, you can track your progress and deepen your understanding of your internal processes.

As highlighted in previous sections, such as the discussion on coping mechanisms, the skills you develop through mindful observation are directly transferable to real-life situations. Over time, you'll find that you have an enhanced capacity to manage stress and emotion, a vital edge in your continuous recovery journey.

Cultivating a mindful approach to challenges

In your sobriety journey, embracing mindfulness is pivotal in significantly enhancing your ability to cope with various challenges. By developing a keen awareness of the present moment, you equip yourself to experience life without the distracting influences of past regrets and future anxieties. By focusing on the now, mindfulness allows you to confront obstacles with a calm and focused mind, thus enabling you to navigate through difficulties with clarity and purpose.

Through mindfulness, you learn to observe your thoughts and emotions without judgment, creating a space between your experiences and your reactions. This gap allows you to choose your response rather than being pulled into impulsive actions or overwhelmed by emotions. Regularly practicing mindfulness builds resilience, allowing you to remain steady and collected even under stress. This resilient mindset is particularly beneficial in sobriety, as it helps you handle triggers and stressors without falling back into addictive patterns.

Embracing the challenges mindfully

In the face of life's inevitable challenges, a mindful approach can be your anchor, keeping you steady and focused. This exercise is designed to help you face difficulties with mindfulness, enabling you to respond with composure and clarity.

You'll need a quiet place where you won't be disturbed; a journal, a digital device, or a piece of paper; and a pen.

Follow these instructions:

1. Prepare:

- Find a quiet space where you can sit comfortably without interruptions.
- Take a few deep breaths to center yourself.

2. Identify a challenge:

- Think of a current challenge you are facing in your sobriety journey.
- Write it down in your journal.

3. Reflect mindfully:

- Close your eyes and reflect on this challenge. What emotions does it evoke? Fear, anxiety, frustration?

4. Breathe through it:

- Focus on your breath, taking slow and deep breaths.
- With each exhale, visualize releasing some of the tension associated with this challenge.

5. Observe your thoughts:

- Pay attention to the thoughts that arise regarding this challenge.
- Imagine these thoughts as clouds passing in the sky, not permanent, just passing through your awareness.

6. Consider mindful responses:

- With a calm mind, consider possible responses to this challenge.
- Write down these responses, focusing on those that promote well-being and recovery.

7. Commit to action:

- Choose a response that feels aligned with your values and commitment to sobriety.
- Write down a plan of action with the steps you will take.

8. Practice regularly:

- Engage in this exercise regularly, especially when new challenges arise.
- Over time, notice any shifts in your ability to handle difficulties with greater ease.

9. Reflect:

- After completing the exercise, take a moment to reflect on the experience. Notice if there's a change in how you perceive the challenge. By practicing mindful engagement with obstacles, you cultivate emotional resilience and a stable foundation for your sobriety.

TIP

Navigating sobriety with mindful resilience in the journey of recovery, consider challenges not as obstacles but as your teachers. To transform difficulties into stepping stones, embrace the pause. When facing a challenge, take a mindful pause. Breathe deeply and give yourself the space to observe your thoughts and feelings without judgment. This pause is a powerful tool — it's your moment of choice where you can respond with intention rather than reacting out of habit.

Research has shown mindfulness to modify brain regions linked with attention and emotional regulation — areas vital for recovery. Practice mindfulness regularly, and you'll strengthen these neural pathways, improving your resilience in the face of challenges.

REMEMBER

Each challenge is an opportunity to reaffirm your commitment to sobriety. By using mindfulness to maintain a steady course, you will survive these trials and emerge stronger and more self-aware. Resilience is like a muscle, and every mindful moment is a rep that makes it stronger.

Mindfulness in the face of your personal sparks

Sparks (triggers) are an inevitable part of recovery, but your response to them doesn't have to be predetermined. By adopting mindfulness, you consciously choose to experience and acknowledge these sparks without judgment. This practice empowers you to recognize the root of your emotional responses and gradually learn to disengage from reflexive, often destructive behaviors. Mindfulness encourages you to observe these triggers as they arise, examining them with curiosity rather than fear. This can help you understand the underlying reasons for your reactions and provide a more stable foundation for dealing with stressors.

Using mindfulness in your daily routine *requires* practice and patience. Start by dedicating a few moments each day to mindful meditation, where you focus solely on your breathing and observe your thoughts and feelings without engagement. This process enhances your ability to act thoughtfully rather than reacting impulsively to sparks. Over time, this training can significantly alter how you respond to challenges, making you more resilient and less likely to turn to unhealthy coping mechanisms.

The journey through recovery is personal and full of various challenges, including external pressures and internal conflicts. Mindfulness equips you with a set of tools that assist in managing these challenges more effectively. By remaining present in the moment, you are better prepared to make choices that align with your long-term goals in sobriety.

REMEMBER

Each moment is an opportunity to practice mindfulness, and each practice is a step toward a more stable and fulfilling life.

FINDING MBSR AND HERSELF WITH JENNY

I've always found solace in the stillness before the day unfolds. I'm an alcoholic, and my name is Jenni. I'm also a stepmom, a wife, a reader, and a member of a bowling team. I'm 15 years into sobriety, and sometimes, it feels like just yesterday when I chose to turn my life around. Yet, as I sit here in the dim light of dawn, a familiar shadow looms, whispering reminders of a job lost and a sense of self not quite found. Honestly, I feel lost again.

My life is full, yet an aching emptiness gnaws at the edges of my days. I have a husband who mirrors my sober journey and two stepchildren who are often the source of both joy and frustration. There's a weight to carrying a role that I never quite auditioned for, and in the silent moments, I'm often left to wrestle with my worthiness.

When I lost my job, the ground beneath me felt unsteady, and the old temptation to pour a glass of wine beckoned like sirens in the distance. I resisted, but the battle left scars, and the triumphant warrior I once saw in the mirror now appeared weary and uncertain.

I found respite in my yoga practice, a place to lay down my burdens with each pose. Meditation became my balm, offering brief reprieves from the relentless chatter of my mind. But the relief was fleeting, like a bandage on a wound that needed stitching. (It was not satisfying!)

It wasn't until I stumbled upon a mindfulness class led by a teacher whose calm seemed as deep as the ocean. There, I found the missing pieces. There, I learned about the Juicy Pause — that sacred space between breaths where I could rest in the present. Selflessness became a lens through which I could see beyond my ego, and open observation allowed me to witness my life without clinging to judgment.

Like lifelines thrown into turbulent waters, these tools helped me still the storm. As I practiced, something within me shifted. The negative self-talk that had been a relentless critic began to lose its power. My thoughts, once dark clouds looming overhead, now drifted by with less menace.

Emboldened by these new strategies, I delved deeper, enrolling in more classes and eventually becoming a guide in MBSR. It was as if I had unlocked a hidden door within myself, revealing a path to peace I didn't know existed.

Most importantly, my heart began to open in ways I couldn't have imagined. The barrier I had unconsciously erected between myself and my stepchildren began to crumble. I found myself cheering at their games with genuine pride, connecting with their youthful challenges, and my husband — my partner in sobriety — now had a wife who could stand beside him, not just in obligation, but in full presence and support.

I am Jenni, sober for 15 years and counting. I am not perfect, nor is my life without its struggles. The voices of doubt whisper less frequently, and the satisfaction of living fully — truly in the moment — is a balm to my once-weary soul.

Integrating mindfulness into daily life for long-term resilience

Incorporating mindfulness into your daily routine involves more than just occasional practice; it's about making it a core component of your daily life. Begin your day with mindful breathing exercises; this simple act can help set a calm tone and awareness for the day ahead. Dedicate moments throughout your day to pause and meditate, even if it's just for a minute or two. These practices help you develop a continuous awareness of your thoughts and emotions, enabling you to manage them more effectively and maintain focus on your present activities.

Over time, mindfulness becomes more than a practice — it transforms into a state of being. As you learn to observe your thoughts without judgment and stay in the present moment, you'll discover a significant shift in how you react to stressful situations. This shift in perception reduces the overwhelming nature of challenges, allowing you to approach them with a more balanced and measured response. This skill is particularly valuable in maintaining sobriety, as it provides a stable mental foundation from which to confront and resolve issues without turning to addictive behaviors.

Integrating mindfulness into your routine can greatly improve your overall quality of life. Regular mindfulness exercises like meditation and mindful walking can enhance physical health by reducing stress and increasing attention span. Internally, you build a resilience that is not easily shaken by external circumstances. Your relationships can also benefit as mindfulness teaches you to listen more deeply and respond more thoughtfully, fostering stronger and more meaningful connections.

REMEMBER

Embed mindfulness into your daily routine, establishing it as a steadfast presence rather than an occasional practice. Start your mornings with deep, mindful breaths to set a tone of awareness, and let that serenity infuse your day with regular pauses for presence. This sustained awareness trains you to observe your thoughts without judgment, enhancing your ability to handle stress calmly, deepening your relationships, and reinforcing your resolve in sobriety.

Mindfulness is not merely a tool to be summoned in times of distress; it is a lifestyle, a continuous thread woven through every hour and minute of your existence. The commitment to start each day with mindful breathing is an invitation to greet the world with equanimity and attentiveness. Sprinkling your day with brief, meditative pauses allows you to sow seeds of peace that will flourish within you.

Here's a possible daily routine that may resonate with your journey:

>> **Morning:**

- Upon waking, engage in a brief mindful breathing session for 5–10 minutes. Focus on the sensation of breath entering and leaving your body.

- Follow this with gentle stretching or yoga to awaken your body, maintaining awareness of your movements and breathing.

- Have a healthy breakfast, taking the time to savor the flavors and textures of your food and practicing mindful eating.

>> **Mid-morning:**

- Take short breaks during work or activities to practice mindful observation. Spend a minute or two to simply notice your surroundings, the sounds, scents, and your inner state without judgment.

- Incorporate mindful walking into your routine, even if it's just a walk from your car to the office. Be present with each step and breath.

>> **Lunchtime:**

- Prioritize a mindful lunch break. Eat away from your desk or work area to minimize distractions and focus on the act of nourishing your body.

- After eating, find a quiet space for a brief midday meditation, using an app or a guided recording if helpful.

>> **Afternoon:**

- Engage in a short aerobic exercise session, like brisk walking or cycling. Use this time to practice awareness of your body's movements and the sensations of exertion, linking this physical activity with mindful presence.

- If you are overwhelmed or stressed, pause for a mindful reset, focusing on your breath to center yourself.

>> **Evening:**

- After work, participate in a more extended exercise session, whether it's a gym workout, a swim, or a run. Treat this time as a moving meditation, observing the thoughts and feelings that arise without getting attached to them.

- Prepare dinner mindfully, paying attention to the colors and textures of the ingredients, the sounds of cooking, and the aromas that fill your kitchen.

>> **Night:**

- As the day winds down, reflect on your day with a gratitude journal or a mindfulness app that can guide you through reflective practices.

- Before bed, engage in some relaxation exercises or guided imagery to help transition into a restful sleep state.

REMEMBER

Your routine can be tailored to fit your individual needs and may evolve over time as you discover the practices that most support your long-term recovery and resilience.

Take these lessons and experiences from this chapter, and let them light your path. May your practice of mindfulness nurture a life of balance, strength, and deep connection — indispensable qualities in your pursuit of lasting sobriety and a life of rich fulfillment.

6

The Part of Tens

Discover your core values to guide your actions in recovery

Create an intentional lifestyle that promotes long-term sobriety

Chapter **16**

Ten Ways to Discover Your Sobriety Purpose

E mbark on your pursuit of purpose in recovery by examining your foundational beliefs and identifying what is of utmost importance to you. These values are the backbone of your decisions and behaviors. Understanding your values helps clarify your path and aligns your actions with your true self, creating a purpose-driven life.

In this chapter, you will explore various strategies to discover your purpose in sobriety, beginning with reflecting on your values. You will learn to set meaningful goals, explore your passions, and connect with others. By being of service, practicing vision exercises, seeking professional guidance, educating yourself, embracing growth, and celebrating wins, you will uncover a fulfilling and purpose-driven life in sobriety. You are now welcome to begin creating a life so good for yourself that you never want to go back to your old way of living.

Set Goals

Setting goals is an important part of structuring your recovery. Divide your goals into small, medium, and long-term goals. Breaking goals into smaller steps helps manage milestones, ensuring you have a clear roadmap. Small goals include daily tasks or weekly objectives, medium goals are monthly achievements, and long-term goals are those you aim to accomplish over a year or more. Each goal achieved brings you a step closer to discovering your fuller, sober self, reinforcing your progress, and boosting your confidence along the way. It's important to enjoy the journey. The destination is a result of the steps you take along the way.

Explore Passions

Rediscover and pursue your passions; these are gateways to fulfillment and joy in sobriety. Think back to interests you've stuffed away because other things became more of a priority or new ones you've wished to explore. Whether it's painting, playing an instrument, writing, gardening, or any other activity that sparks your curiosity, dive back into it. Actively engaging in your passions can rekindle joy and give a newfound purpose to your life. These activities provide a healthy distraction and allow you to connect with your authentic self, bringing excitement and meaning to your sober journey.

Connect with Others

Create and build connections with others who share similar journeys or values. Your interactions can provide support, exchange experiences, and offer new perspectives, which are helpful when navigating sobriety. Seek support groups, attend meetings, or join clubs and communities that align with your interests and values. These connections can deepen your understanding of yourself and others, fostering a sense of belonging and camaraderie. As you share your struggles and wins, you'll find encouragement and motivation, making the path to sobriety feel less lonely and more manageable. Allow others to offer you that safe space to be you.

Service to Others

Service is a profound way to find purpose. This could be through volunteering, participating in outreach programs, or simple acts like talking to someone who is going through a hard time. Service shifts focus from self to others, enriching your sense of purpose while helping others. Volunteering at local shelters, mentoring those new to sobriety, or even helping out at community events are excellent ways to give back. These acts of kindness make a huge difference in the lives of others but also enhance your journey by building a sense of connection, empathy, and fulfillment.

Practice Vision Exercises

Create and regularly practice vision exercises to visualize your future self. Picture yourself as already having achieved your goals and embodying your true values. Imagine the life you want to live and then spend a few minutes each day imagining yourself already having achieved it, focusing on the positive changes you've made and successes you've had. Visualize yourself overcoming challenges, celebrating milestones, and living in alignment with your core values. Visualizing a successful recovery can be incredibly motivating, helping you manifest your aspirations into reality. By clearly seeing your desired future, you reinforce your commitment and inspire yourself to take actionable steps toward making that vision a reality.

Seek Professional Guidance

Don't hesitate to seek professional advice. Coaches and counselors can provide valuable guidance, help refine your strategies, and offer feedback to enhance your recovery and keep it pointing toward an amazing future. Engaging with professionals enriches your journey with expert insights. They can help you identify potential obstacles, develop effective coping mechanisms, and set realistic, achievable goals. Regular sessions with a professional can also provide accountability, ensuring you stay on track. Whether individual counseling, group therapy, or life coaching, their support can offer a fresh perspective and additional support, making your path to sobriety smoother and more successful.

Educate Yourself

Continuous learning is essential. Educate yourself about addiction, recovery strategies, and personal development. Read books, attend workshops, or take online courses to expand your knowledge. Learning new things enlightens and empowers you, providing tools to manage challenges and advance in your sobriety. Understanding the science behind addiction and our brains and gaining insights into self-improvement can contribute to a stronger, more resilient you. The more you know, the better equipped you are to navigate your journey and maintain a healthy, fulfilling, sober life.

Embrace Growth

Step outside your comfort zone and embrace growth because that is where the *magic* of life happens. Long-term recovery requires adapting to changes and trying new ways of living. Embracing these changes can significantly impact self-discovery and personal growth within your sober life. Try new things, meet new people, and explore different environments. Challenge yourself to do things that might have seemed too hard or daunting before.

Each new experience can teach you something valuable and help you grow stronger. By stepping into the unknown, you open up possibilities for a more fulfilling life in sobriety.

Celebrate Wins

Always take time to celebrate your wins, no matter how small they might appear. Acknowledge and enjoy your achievements; these are important milestones in your recovery. Celebrations reinforce positive behaviors and remind you of your abilities to overcome challenges in pursuit of long-term sobriety. Each victory is worth recognizing. Treat yourself to something special, share your success with loved ones, or take a moment to reflect on your progress. Celebrating your wins boosts your confidence and motivates you to keep moving forward on your journey.

As you come to the end of this chapter, discovering your purpose in sobriety is a continuous, evolving journey. Each step brings you closer to a life filled with meaning and fulfillment. Embrace the strategies shared here, and let them guide you toward a deeper understanding of yourself and your place in the world. Celebrate your progress, no matter how small, and keep pushing forward with determination and hope. Your journey to a purpose-driven, sober life is uniquely yours, and every effort you make is a testament to your strength and resilience. Keep moving forward, and know that the best is yet to come.

Navigate Social Situations and Awkwardness

Sobriety is a courageous journey that doesn't end with putting down the drink; it extends into every aspect of your daily life, including the complex puzzle of social interactions. By seeking the warmth of a supportive community, finding company in a sober companion, or indulging in non-alcoholic activities, you reinforce your sobriety while navigating social terrains.

While your sobriety journey may shift your social landscape, it also opens the door to genuine connection and self-discovery. Challenges will inevitably arise as you navigate events and environments steeped in alcohol culture. Still, with a supportive network and a roster of sober activities, each social interaction becomes an opportunity for growth. Embrace your sober identity with confidence, knowing that the strategies you build — finding a sober companion, engaging in new hobbies, and seeking professional guidance — will transform these challenges into stepping stones for a rewarding and resilient sober life.

Chapter **17**

Ten Ways to Achieve Long-Term Sobriety

N ow that you're on sobriety journey, finding ways to avoid having it derailed is critical. You've come a long way, so use these tips to help stay on your journey, achieving long-term sobriety.

Find a Sense of Connection

Cultivating a strong sense of connection is crucial in your recovery, as it helps overcome resistance and fear. This involves introspective work to understand the beliefs driving your actions and healing. Spirituality can also provide grounding and values that support your commitment to sobriety. However, the primary focus is on the impact of interpersonal relationships, which serve as pillars in your recovery journey. Engaging with a supportive community, such as recovery groups or sober networks, can offer invaluable mutual support and understanding. These connections provide a safety net and enrich your support network during challenging times. Regular involvement in shared activities or online forums allows you to exchange stories, offer advice, and receive encouragement, fostering a sense of belonging and shared purpose. Nurturing healthy friendships that support sobriety is essential. These relationships help build a strong foundation for your recovery, offering companionship and accountability. Whether through regular meetings, shared activities, or mentorship, a robust support system fortifies your recovery by providing diverse perspectives and collective strength.

"Connection is fundamental to our sense of security and safety. Through relationships with ourselves, our beliefs, our values, others, and the broader world, we learn to feel comfortable and secure."

–Ellen E. Elliott, PhD, LCAS, LCMHC, CCS, CSAT

Build a Strong Community

Building a strong community means stepping out of isolation and surrounding yourself with people who support your journey. It involves proactively seeking out and engaging with individuals and groups who understand the challenges of addiction and the importance of recovery. Whether through recovery meetings, support groups, or social networks dedicated to sobriety, connecting with others who share similar goals can provide the encouragement and accountability necessary to maintain your commitment. These relationships offer emotional support during tough times, celebrate your milestones, and provide practical advice based on shared experiences.

"Recovery community organizations (RCOs) are vital for sustained sobriety, offering peer support, education, and advocacy for those in recovery from substance use disorders. These peer-led nonprofits host recovery meetings and support groups, provide educational workshops on relapse prevention and stress management, and promote sober social activities to build a sense of community. RCOs focus on empowerment, outreach, and reducing the stigma around recovery."

–Ashley Sunderland, BA, CPP, LADC, CPRS

Get Professional Help/Support

Building a strong community means stepping out of isolation and surrounding yourself with people who support your journey. This involves proactively seeking out and engaging with individuals and groups who understand the challenges of addiction and the importance of recovery. Whether through recovery meetings, support groups, or social networks dedicated to sobriety, connecting with others who share similar goals can provide the encouragement and accountability necessary to maintain your commitment. These relationships offer emotional support during tough times, celebrate your milestones, and provide practical advice based on shared experiences. By surrounding yourself with a robust and supportive network, you create an environment where recovery is possible, sustainable, and enriching.

"Informed consent is vital in addiction recovery, extending beyond initial information at intake. It's an ongoing dialogue ensuring you fully understand any treatment's risks and benefits. Quality care should empower you to make decisions aligned with your sobriety goals and well-being. Your health is paramount, and your informed consent should always be prioritized."

–Jeffrey Quamme, MS, AADC, CCS, CNE, CNC, chief executive officer at www.ctcertboard.org

Design Your Life of Sobriety

Designing your sober lifestyle is an intentional act of reinvention. Your foundation is built upon routines and habits that celebrate and sustain a life free from alcohol. This involves a thoughtful composition of your daily activities, relationships, and personal endeavors, all collectively supporting long-term sobriety. Designing your sober life means curating a vibrant and rewarding existence where happiness comes from clarity and purpose. It involves making deliberate choices about how you spend your time, who you surround yourself with, and what personal goals you strive to achieve. Rediscover joy in simple moments, excitement in new challenges, and peace in serenity. This journey of self-rediscovery and reinvention leads to a profoundly fulfilling and balanced life, where your sobriety serves as a cornerstone for continuous personal growth and happiness.

"Recovery is a launching pad. Over many years, I've found that no matter the circumstances, there can always be greater emotional sobriety. There is always a next level of progress. Never stop exploring ways to grow. Every difficulty contains the seeds of transformation."

—Ronald Chapman, founder of ProgressiveRecovery.org, author of *Progressive Recovery Through the Twelve Steps: Emotionally Sober for Life*

Develop Coping Skills

It's crucial to develop new coping skills to replace the old ones that involve addiction. Your previous methods of dealing with stress, disappointment, and even celebration may have revolved around drinking or other addictive behaviors. To maintain long-term sobriety and prevent relapse, finding healthier and more constructive ways to handle these emotions is essential. This starts with identifying the specific sparks that lead you to seek solace in addiction and then consciously choosing alternative strategies that offer genuine relief without harmful consequences. Engaging in physical activities such as exercise, yoga, or regular walks can provide an excellent outlet for stress relief and emotional regulation, releasing endorphins that lift your mood. By developing a robust set of coping mechanisms, you equip yourself with the tools necessary to navigate life's ups and downs without falling back into old, destructive habits, thereby protecting your sobriety and enhancing your overall quality of life.

"In your recovery journey, find a 'workout buddy' in your support network — someone you trust who understands sobriety challenges. Be kind to yourself; use pen and paper to release anxious thoughts and stay present. Define your spiritual health based on your purpose."

—Scott Gorman, professional sports recovery consultant at firmarecovery.com

Keep Learning

On the path to sobriety, learning never stops. Knowledge is a powerful tool in your recovery arsenal, soIn the path to sobriety, the learning never stops. Knowledge is a powerful tool in your recovery arsenal, keep learning., keep learning.

In the path to sobriety, the learning never stops. Knowledge is a powerful tool in your recovery arsenal. Continuously educating yourself about the nature of addiction, the psychological and physiological effects of substance abuse, and the latest research on effective recovery strategies can empower you to make informed decisions about your health and well-being. Attending workshops, reading books, and participating in online courses or support groups can expand your understanding and provide new insights and techniques for managing your sobriety. This commitment to lifelong learning keeps you engaged in your recovery process and helps you stay adaptable and resilient in the face of challenges. By staying curious and open to new information, you can continually refine and strengthen your approach to living a sober, fulfilling life.

"Never stop learning, improving, or believing. To keep learning is to stay humble and open to the unknown, allowing new insights to transform my perspective. Learning is a lifelong journey; our purpose is to explore, learn, and grow."

—Murphy Jensen, recovery mentor, founder of WEconnect.com,
French Open champion, cardiac arrest survivor,
and mental health advocate

Set goals for Long-Term Recovery

Your journey to long-term recovery is a deeply personal endeavor, yet it benefits immensely from the collective strength of a community that understands exactly what you're going through. Surrounding yourself with like-minded individuals committed to sobriety provides a valuable support system where you can share experiences, challenges, and successes. These connections offer empathy, encouragement, and accountability, helping you stay motivated and focused on your recovery goals. Whether through support groups, therapy sessions, or informal gatherings, being part of a community that shares your commitment to a sober lifestyle can foster a sense of belonging and reduce feelings of isolation.

"Thriving in recovery means unlocking your potential and taking steps toward your best life daily. Never lose hope, document your goals, and seek a reliable support network. With honesty, self-love, and commitment, you can overcome addiction and transform your life."

–POP Buchanan, founder of Sober is Dope, author, recording artist, NFT artist, and owner of Grand Echelon Records

Change Your Lifestyle

Finding yourself is the most significant change in your sober life, opening the door to endless possibilities. As you eliminate alcohol from your life, you will constantly be invited to explore new facets of who you are and the world around you. Instead of checking out, you become present, fully engaging with your emotions, surroundings, and relationships. This shift allows you to experience life more profoundly and authentically. The initial overwhelming brightness of sobriety gradually softens into a warm glow, illuminating your path of self-discovery and personal growth. Living without the need for numbing agents means embracing the full range of human emotions — joy, sadness, uncertainty, and anger — as integral parts of your experience. By changing just one thing — removing alcohol — you set off a ripple effect that transforms your entire life, leading to a more fulfilling and nurturing existence grounded in authenticity and meaning.

"Long-term sobriety often involves significant lifestyle changes, such as maintaining a well-fed brain."

–Christina Veselak, MS, LMFT, CN

Practice mindfulness and Meditation

As discussed in several chapters, mindfulness and meditation are crucial tools for understanding and developing a relationship with your sober life. By practicing mindfulness, you can enhance your emotional regulation, improve your ability to cope with stress and build resilience against triggers that may lead to relapse. Clinical studies have shown that mindfulness-based stress reduction (MBSR) can significantly reduce the use of substances and improve overall mental health. Mindfulness helps increase gray matter concentration in areas of the brain related to learning, memory, and emotion regulation, which are particularly beneficial in navigating cravings and maintaining long-term sobriety. Simple practices such as deep breathing, mindful observation, and progressive relaxation can easily integrate into your daily routine, providing a mental buffer against stressors.

"Mindfulness is a powerful practice that significantly aids all stages of sobriety by addressing core symptoms of addiction such as craving, impulsivity, negative mood, and stress. It reshapes the brain to improve focus, mood, and empathy while reducing distractions and stress. This practice builds resilience, serenity, and compassion, making it invaluable for maintaining long-term sobriety and overall well-being."

–Gus Castellanos, MD

Explore mental Health/ Medication

Proper mental health care and appropriate medication can be crucial components of your recovery journey, playing a significant role in stabilizing your mood, reducing symptoms of anxiety and depression, and supporting your overall well-being. Addressing underlying mental health issues is often essential for effective long-term recovery, as these conditions can be both a cause and a consequence of substance abuse. Working with healthcare professionals, such as therapists, psychiatrists, and counselors, can provide you with a comprehensive treatment plan tailored to your specific needs. Medications such as antidepressants, anti-anxiety drugs, or mood stabilizers may be prescribed to help manage symptoms and create a stable foundation for your recovery efforts. Therapy modalities like cognitive-behavioral therapy (CBT), dialectical behavior therapy (DBT), and other evidence-based approaches can complement medication by providing strategies to cope with stress, change negative thought patterns, and build healthier habits.

"Being proactive about your mental health — by staying informed about treatments, being honest with yourself and your providers, and incorporating practices like mindfulness and exercise — can significantly enhance your quality of life. Prioritizing mental well-being lays a strong foundation for lasting recovery and a fulfilling, addiction-free life."

–Jeffrey Quamme, CEO Connecticut Certification Board, Inc., http://www.ctcertboard.org

Index

A

AA (Alcoholics Anonymous), 11, 19, 20, 57, 62

accountability, peer support and, 65

ACEs (adverse childhood experiences), 99, 100–101

acknowledging impact of substance abuse, 26

actions
  for long-term sobriety, 281
  ownership of, 40

activities, identifying, 198–200

activity zones, 287

adaptability, science of in goal-setting, 80

addiction
  cross-addictions, 14–16
  as a family disease, 250–251
  growth of, 11–13
  mechanisms of, 93

advanced classes, in years 6–15 of sobriety, 71

advanced educational pursuits, in years 16+ of sobriety, 72

adventure sports, in years 6–15 of sobriety, 71

adverse childhood experiences (ACEs), 99, 100–101

alcohol use, glorification of, 12

alcohol use disorder. See alcoholism

alcoholic, heavy drinker compared with, 13–14

Alcoholics Anonymous (AA), 11, 19, 20, 57, 62

alcoholism
  about, 10–11
  growth of, 11–13

aligning career goals, with sobriety, 262–263

alternatives
  designing healthier, 32
  treatments, 167–170

amino acids, 181–182, 300

amygdala, 161

ancestral narrative exploration, 226

anchoring recovery, in positive habits, 226

anger
  healthy response strategies to, 47
  unhealthy response strategies to, 45

anterior cingulate cortex, 161

anxiety
  healthy response strategies to, 47
  managing, 164–166
  unhealthy response strategies to, 45

appendices, in relapse prevention plan, 239

art exhibitions, in years 16+ of sobriety, 72

art therapy, in years 1–5 of sobriety, 71

aspirations, personal and professional, 214–215

assertiveness
  of saying "no," 144–145
  training, as a healthy coping mechanism, 285

awkwardness, 361–362

Ayahuasca, 169

B

balancing
  social connections, 210
  work and leisure in recovery, 69–72

U

unresolved issues, 115

V

Veselak, Christina, 368
victories, celebrating small, 29
vision exercises, practicing, 359
volunteering
  as a healthy coping mechanism, 285
  in years 1-5 of sobriety, 71
vulnerability
  embracing, 40
  as a strength, 57–58

W

walking meditation, 334
Warning icon, 6

warning signs, identifying, 287–291
well-being. *See specific types*
Wellbriety, 19
willingness, as a spiritual principle
  for long-term recovery, 121
Wilson, Bill (AA founder), 171
wins, celebrating, 361
work, balancing with leisure in
  recovery, 69–72
work events, 273–274
workplace support systems, 274

Y

yoga, in years 1-5 of sobriety, 71

About the Authors

Lane Kennedy is a person living in long-term recovery. Not *just* a mindfulness and meditation teacher; she's a force of nature in the world of personal wellness. With a deep passion for helping people find equilibrium in their lives, she leverages her expertise as a functional DNA nutritionist to guide individuals toward long-term health. Lane believes that *listening* and mindfulness should be a core part of the curriculum in grade school, alongside nutrition, to foster healthier, more empathetic communities.

Her love for heritage apples and her habit of drinking lots of water reflect her commitment to a balanced lifestyle. Lane also doesn't believe in complaining; instead, she advocates for taking proactive action in one's life. Although her desk may accumulate piles over time, she knows exactly where everything is and appreciates a good reorganization session every few months, often needing a phone call or a companion to assist.

Over the past five years, Lane has made significant contributions to the wellness program provided by the City of San Francisco, serving approximately 40,000 employees as their mindfulness teacher. She has created and facilitated meditation, breath work, and mindfulness classes for city employees, including first responders. These classes are essential for helping them regulate their nervous systems during high-stress situations.

She is an ardent fan of classic rock and loves a good round of "name that tune."

Tamar Medford was born in 1976 in the Netherlands, and her family immigrated to Canada when she was just one year old. Raised by two wonderful parents who always encouraged her to be her best, Tamar carried those lessons into adulthood. Her father, who has become her hero, modeled a way of living that emphasized the importance of following one's passion, no matter how tough life gets. This philosophy was central to their collaborative effort in creating their first documentary, "Beyond Recovery."

Tamar enjoys taking drives in her Jeep, cranking up the music, and feeling the freedom of the open road. She also loves a good games night with her partner, the kids, and friends. Though most of her family remains overseas, she has made Canada her home. As a long-term goal, she dreams of purchasing a home on a white sandy beach in a tropical paradise.

Her unique background and life experiences enrich her contributions to the field of recovery coaching, where she supports individuals in achieving lasting sobriety. Tamar combines her corporate experience and personal development skills to offer pragmatic and supportive guidance, focusing on practical strategies for overcoming the challenges of addiction recovery.

As a podcast producer, Tamar loves bringing people's visions and missions to life, transforming ideas into captivating audio experiences. Her passion for storytelling and connection shines through in every project she undertakes, creating an inspiring platform for voices that need to be heard.

Author's Acknowledgments

First and foremost, we want to extend a huge, heartfelt thanks to Wiley Publishing for its unwavering commitment to individuals seeking answers to all their questions. Working with Wiley has been an absolute breeze—they've been with us every step of the way, ensuring that our vision came to life with ease and support. *If only assembling IKEA furniture were this smooth!*

A huge shout-out to our families, who gifted us hours upon hours of uninterrupted time to create, write, draft, and complete this book. Their patience is nothing short of saintly, and without their support, this endeavor would have been relegated to the land of half-finished projects!

We owe a debt of gratitude to Bill Wilson and the first 100 for creating *"a design for living that really works"* and the vast, open-minded community that embraces the many pathways of recovery. Your pioneering spirits have guided us more than you'll ever know.

A special thank you to The Sober Curator and every single curator who meticulously put together stories and supported our journey in writing. You've been our backbone. And speaking of backbones, Alysse Bryson deserves a standing ovation for being our biggest cheerleader—her enthusiasm is contagious and her belief in us is unshakable.

We are immensely grateful for the myriad of introductions, emails, and Zoom calls that helped shape this book. Special mentions go to Jaclyn Brown, Scott Gorman, Al Cotton, Jeffrey Quame, Murphy Jensen, Cal Beyer, Carolyn Delaney, Emily Feinstein, and so many more. Your contributions have been invaluable, and we've learned so much through this collaborative effort.

Our deepest appreciation also goes to the scientific research teams and communities that tirelessly commit to finding solutions to the disease of alcoholism. To the researchers and the mindfulness community, including Joseph Goldstein, Judson Brewer, Gus Castellanos, your work is nothing short of revolutionary. We are grateful to the endless procession of teachers, guides, recovery guides, treatment teams, and recovery advocates who show up every day to practice whole-body living without drugs and alcohol.

Finally, to you, our reader, who is seeking a better life and embarking on the continuous journey of long-term recovery. Our biggest hope for you is that you learn, enjoy this book, further your knowledge, and have fun in your future sober life. You've got this! Cheers to the collective effort and the beautiful journey of recovery we share!

Publisher's Acknowledgments

Acquisitions Editor: Tracy Boggier

Project Manager: Rick Kughen

Development Editor: Rick Kughen

Technical Editor: Joe Bush

Production Editor: Saikarthick Kumarasamy

Cover Image: © Leonardo Castano/ 500px/Getty Images